John Nielson

Handbook of Contact Dermatitis

Handbook of Contact Dermatitis

Edited by

Matthias Gebhardt MD
Private Dermatology Practice
Zwickau, Germany

Peter Elsner MD
Professor of Dermatology
Friedrich Schiller University
Jena, Germany

and

James G Marks Jr, MD
Professor of Medicine
Section of Dermatology
Pennsylvania State University College of Medicine
Hershey, USA

MARTIN DUNITZ

First published in the United Kingdom in 2000
by Martin Dunitz Ltd, The Livery House, 7–9 Pratt Street, London NW1 0AE

A CIP record for this book is available from the British Library.

ISBN 1-85317-801-2

Distributed in the USA by:
Blackwell Science Inc.
Commerce Place, 350 Main Street
Malden, MA 02148, USA
Tel: 1-800-215-1000

Distributed in Canada by:
Login Brothers Book Company
324 Salteaux Crescent
Winnipeg, Manitoba, R3J 3T2
canada
Tel: 204-224-4068

Distributed in Brazil by:
Ernesto Reichmann Distribuidora de Livros, Ltda
Rua Coronel Marques 335, Tatuape 03440-000
Sao Paulo,
Brazil

Composition by Scribe Design, Gillingham, Kent
Printed and bound in Singapore by Kyodo Printing Co (S'pore) Pte Ltd

Contents

List of Contributors

Ute Barta MD
University Hospital of Freidrich–Schiller University
Department of Dermatology
Jena
Germany

Andrea Bauer MD
University Hospital of Freidrich–Schiller University
Department of Dermatology
Jena
Germany

Undine Berndt MD
University Hospital of Freidrich–Schiller University
Department of Dermatology
Jena
Germany

Peter Elsner MD
University Hospital of Freidrich–Schiller University
Department of Dermatology
Jena
Germany

Matthias Gebhardt MD
Private Dermatology Practice
Zwickau
Germany

Uta–Christina Hipler DSc
University Hospital of Freidrich–Schiller University
Department of Dermatology
Jena
Germany

Dimiter Iliev MD
Ernst von Bergmann Clinic
Department of Dermatology
Postdam
Germany

Theodor Karamfilow MD
University Hospital of Freidrich–Schiller University
Department of Dermatology
Jena
Germany

Annett Looks MD
University Hospital of Freidrich–Schiller University
Department of Dermatology
Jena
Germany

James G Marks Jr, MD
Pennsylvania State University College of Medicine
Section of Dermatology
Hershey
USA

Walter Wigger–Alberti MD
University Hospital of Freidrich–Schiller University
Department of Dermatology
Jena
Germany

Uwe Wollina MD
University Hospital of Freidrich–Schiller University
Department of Dermatology
Jena
Germany

PREFACE

At first sight, contact dermatitis seems to be a frequent and trivial skin disease; however, whilst it is correct that contact dermatitis is frequent in terms of incidence and prevalence, it certainly is not a trivial condition. Its pathogenesis has been a matter for extensive research over the last decades and has provided enormous insight into the complicated mechanisms of the human immune system in general, and not only for skin-related immune reactions. The diagnosis and treatment of the condition require detective skills, huge clinical experience and a trusting interaction between physician and patient, especially in the complicated situations of chronic, recalcitrant contact dermatitis.

Although this wealth of information has been accumulated on the topic of contact dermatitis, in journal publications and excellent textbooks, much of this literature has not reached the general physician or even the general dermatologist in practice. This is a deplorable situation in view of the fact that most contact dermatitis patients are cared for by primary physicians without ever attending a specialized clinic.

The editors therefore thought it to be a timely undertaking to write a short handbook on contact dermatitis, gathering the essentials in the field without confusing the reader with too many details only of interest to the specialists. Obviously, this means taking hard decisions over what is important and what may be omitted; we know that these decisions may be controversial in many cases, but we relied on our common sense sharpened by the daily encounter with contact dermatitis patients. Readers looking for more detailed information are invited to consult the excellent "big" textbooks in the field. We are confident the majority of our readership will appreciate this concise format as useful for their practical purposes.

This project would not have been possible without our colleagues from the Department of Dermatology, Friedrich Schiller University of Jena, who shared their experience as authors and coauthors. Their engagement is gratefully acknowledged. Finally, we would like to thank Dr Sibylle Schliemann-Willers for her extensive editorial support and Yasmin Khan-Chowdhury and Robert Peden of Martin Dunitz Publishers for their kind help with this project.

Matthias Gebhardt
Peter Elsner
James G Marks

1. Introduction: Trends in Contact Dermatitis

Peter Elsner

The skin is one of the most important barrier organs of the human body, protecting internal homeostasis (water, minerals, temperature) and protecting the body from harmful environmental influences. It is constantly exposed to physical, chemical and biological environmental factors. As soon as the damage induced by these factors exceeds the tolerance and repair capacity of the skin, disease will occur. Physical pressure may cause ulcers, UV radiation may cause sunburn, chemicals may cause dermatitis or urticaria, and biological organisms may cause infection. Thus, dermatology is broadly a specialty of environmental medicine, although individuals' thresholds for disease certainly vary according to genetic disposition.

Contact dermatitis is a specific environmental skin disease, an inflammatory skin reaction to noxious agents in the environment. This disease is not characterized by the causative agent, but by the typical morphology of the inflammatory reaction, which is called "eczematous". While in the chronic forms of contact dermatitis the clinical signs are rather unspecific, signs of the acute forms may be more characteristic depending on the disease mechanism: irritant or allergic.

In acute irritant contact dermatitis (ICD) a sharply demarcated erythema, oedema, bullae and possibly necrosis can be found, whereas in acute allergic contact dermatitis (ACD) the borders of the lesions are typically blurred, and erythema, papules and vesicles are present (Figure 1.1). These primary lesions are consistently followed by erosions, oozing, crusting and desquamation, a time-related typical sequence of events ("metachronic polymorphia").

In chronic ICD and ACD it is typical that many lesions are present at the same time ("synchronic polymorphia"): in addition to those already mentioned, lichenification (inflammatory thickening of the skin which frequently results in painful cracking and fissures), hyperkeratosis and desquamation may be found. The subjective symptoms of contact dermatitis are itch, which is sometimes severe, and (mainly in ACD) burning and pain. In chronic cases of contact dermatitis of the hands and feet, pain due to fissures can be severe and disabling.

The two types of contact dermatitis, ICD and ACD, while frequently clinically indistinguishable, are clearly different from a pathogenetic perspective. ICD is induced by non-specific toxicants that damage epidermal and/or dermal structures. Anyone may develop ICD, depending on their individual threshold, and the disease shows a monophasic pattern: damage followed by repair. In contrast, ACD requires a genetic predisposition to develop a specific Th1-cell response to

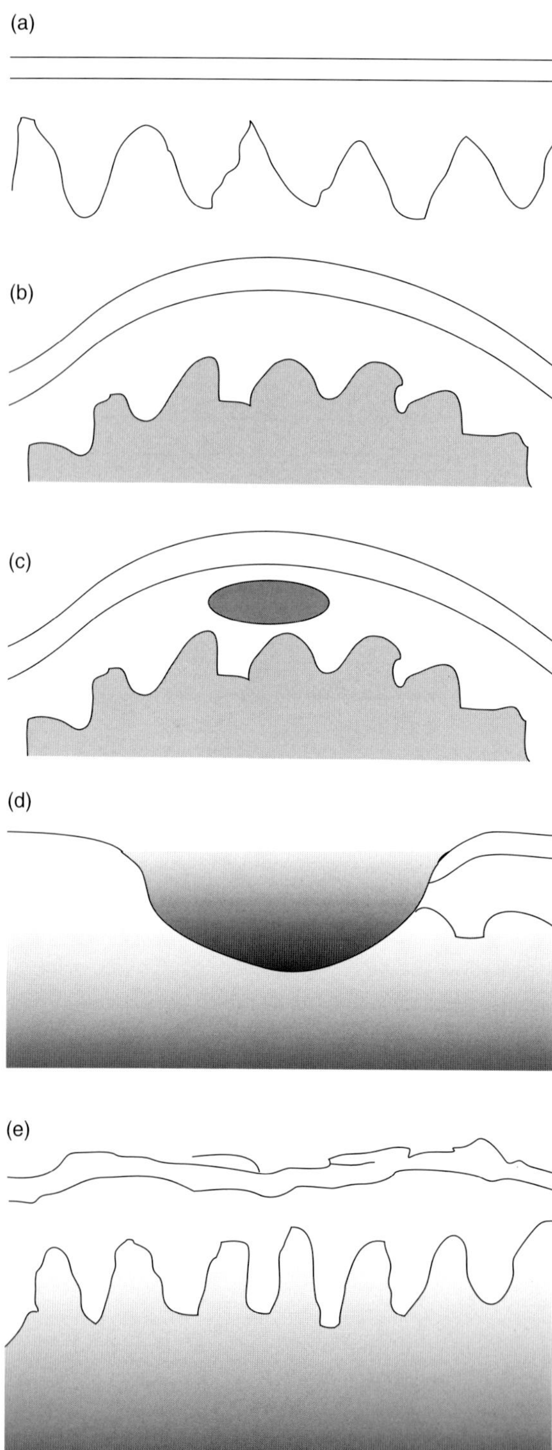

Figure 1.1: Lesions of contact dermatitis: a, normal skin; b, papule; c, papulovesicle; d, excoriation and crusting; e, lichenification and desquamation.

a given allergen, and the disease is biphasic: an induction phase is followed by an elicitation phase. Therefore, on first contact with an allergen, allergic dermatitis may develop only after a silent period of approximately 2 weeks. It is a hypersensitivity disease, i.e. an allergen dose that is completely innocuous to the unsensitized may cause intensive dermatitic reactions in sensitized individuals. While the basic disease pattern for ICD and ACD is different, recent research has shown that later events such as expression of cytokines and adhesion molecules in the skin, leading to cell damage and attraction of inflammatory cells, are highly comparable between the two entities.

Because ICD and ACD cannot be differentiated with certainty on clinical grounds, patch testing remains an essential tool in the diagnostic process. Introduced by Josef Jadassohn as early as 1895, the principle remains unchanged despite technical improvements. Basically, allergens in a non-irritant dose are applied on healthy skin under occlusion, thus deliberately inducing ACD in the sensitized. Only if exposure to an allergen, consequent disease and positive patch test to the allergen are concordant, can ACD be diagnosed. No test procedures exist for the diagnosis of ICD. Therefore, ICD is always diagnosed by an exclusion method, i.e. negative patch tests to allergens with which the patient had been in contact. In practice, this frequently leaves doubt, because allergen exposure may have been unnoticed and thus allergens may be missed in the patch testing work-up.

It is with these limitations in mind that epidemiological figures on the prevalence and incidence of contact dermatitis have to be viewed. Estimates of contact dermatitis in the general population vary between 2 and 11%.[1] However, population-based epidemiological studies frequently lack the detailed work-up described above, and they therefore group all dermatitis cases together, e.g. including atopic hand dermatitis and contact dermatitis. It is important to remember that contact dermatitis frequently is a relapsing disease. Therefore, point prevalence that only registers the actual cases at a given time point is typically much lower than period prevalence, i.e. the addition of cases over a time period. In a Swedish study, the point prevalence of hand dermatitis in a city population was reported to be 5.4%, whereas the 1-year period prevalence was 10.6%.[2] Incidence rates of contact dermatitis were rarely investigated. In Germany, where cases of occupational dermatitis have to be reported, a population-based study showed 3-year incidence rates per 10,000 employees as being between 580 for hairdressers and 25 for leather workers.[1] With the current scarcity of data, however, it is impossible to judge with any certainty whether the incidence and prevalence of contact dermatitis have changed in recent years.

Certainly, the spectrum of allergens that are reported in multicentre studies shows characteristic time-related changes in the Western world. Such allergens now have a reduced frequency in many populations, such as potassium dichromate (due to decreased direct skin contact of construction workers with concrete), while others have increased, such as the fragrance mix (probably reflecting increased exposure to perfumed cosmetics and household products). In a recent German multicentre study of 40,000 patients, population-adjusted frequencies of sensitization for the four most frequent allergens were nickel sulphate 12.9%, fragrance mix 10.5%, balsam of Peru 7.3%, and thimerosal 5.6%.[3] Despite attempts to prevent the introduction of new allergens in cosmetics, household products and in the occupational setting by structure–activity relationship analysis and predictive testing in animal assays, there is an increasing number of new chemical substances introduced into the environment and it is safe to predict the constant detection of new allergens causing contact dermatitis in consumers and workers.[4] Hopefully preventive measures, such as the banning of fashion jewellery releasing nickel into the skin in allergy-eliciting amounts, will reduce the overall incidence and prevalence of contact dermatitis in the future.[5]

References

1. Diepgen TL, Coenraads PJ, Inflammatory skin dieases II: contact dermatitis. In: Williams HC, Strachan DP, eds. *The challenge of dermatoepidemiology*. Boca Raton: CRC Press, 1997: 145–161.

2. Meding B, Swanbeck G, Occupational hand eczema in an industrial city. *Contact Dermatitis* 1990; **22**:13–23.

3. Schnuch A, Geier J, Uter W et al., National rates and regional differences in sensitization to allergens of the standard series. Population-adjusted frequencies of sensitization (PAFS) in 40,000 patients from a multicenter study (IVDK). *Contact Dermatitis* 1997; **37**:200–209.

4. Barker MO, Newer cosmetic ingredients – new patch testing problems? *Am J Contact Dermatitis* **9**:130–135.

5. Menne T, Prevention of nickel allergy by regulation of specific exposures. *Ann Clin Lab Sci* 1996; **26**:133–138.

2. Immunopathology of Allergic and Irritant Contact Dermatitis

Uwe Wollina

Contact dermatitis is common and is the most common job-related disease of the Western world. Its nature can be either irritant or allergic. On the basis of clinical observations or histological examination, the two cannot be clearly distinguished. However, their immunopathology seems to be different.

Allergic contact dermatitis

Allergic contact dermatitis (ACD) starts with sensitization. In general, the hapten or antigen is encountered epicutaneously, but haematogenic sensitization may occur in rare cases. Following penetration of the skin, haptens or antigens are taken up by epidermal Langerhans cells, which process them and migrate to the regional lymph nodes. There, the antigen is presented to naïve T cells. The Langerhans cells must be activated either by the hapten itself or by keratinocyte-derived proinflammatory cytokines. The activated Langerhans cell is capable of secreting various cytokines (interleukins: IL-1β, IL-6, IL-12, etc.) and expresses cell surface molecules (MHC I and II, adhesion molecules, etc.). Other co-migratory factors for Langerhans cells are tumour necrosis factor α (TNF-α) and the granulocyte–macrophage colony-stimulating factor (GM-CSF). It is apparent that Langerhans cells play a crucial role in the sensitization process but other antigen-presenting cells (APCs) such as dermal dendritic cells, may also contribute to the priming of naïve T cells.

Hapten presentation to naïve T cells results in activation and generation of not only T-effector but also T-suppressor cells. Most haptens/antigens evoke an oligoclonal T-cell response consisting mainly of CD8+ cells. The ratio of effector/suppressor cells depends upon the hapten dose; lowering the dose may result in tolerance induction (Table 2.1).

The elicitation phase of ACD is characterized by mast cell degranulation, vasodilatation, and migration of neutrophils, mononuclear cells and T cells. It has been assumed that antigen-specific primed T cells patrol the skin and flares of ACD are elicited when these cells encounter the relevant antigen presented by epidermal Langerhans cells. This view has been questioned, however, because the number of intraepidermal T cells is rather low and they may not provide a

Table 2.1 Dose-dependent T-cell response during antigen presentation (according to Grabbe & Schwarz[2])

Antigen dosage	*Cells presenting antigen*	*T-cell response*		
High	Langerhans cells and others	Optimally primed T effector cells, inadequately primed T suppressor cells	→	Contact hypersensitivity
Lower	Langerhans cells alone	T Effector cells alone	→	Contact hypersensitivity
Very low	Langerhans cells and others	Inadequately primed T suppressor cells	→	Low-zone tolerance

Table 2.2 Differences between ACD and other types of delayed-type hypersensitivity (modified after Enk[1] and Grabbe & Schwarz[2])

	Allergic contact dermatitis	*Delayed-type hypersensitivity*
MHC restriction	MHC I & II	MHC II
Effector T lymphocytes	CD8 (Tc1), CD4 (Th1, Th2), γδ T cells	CD4 (Th1)
Negative regulatory cells		
Conventional sensitization	CD4 (Th2)	CD8
Low-zone tolerance	CD8	?
Cytokines		
Sensitization	IL-1β, IL-12	IL-12
Elicitation	IL-1, IL-4, IL-12, TNF-α, IFN-γ	IL-1, IL-8, IL-12, TNF-α, IFN-γ

sufficient response. Furthermore, activated Langerhans cells emigrate from the epidermis into lymph nodes; these cells could not be available for intraepidermal T cells. Finally, the hapten-induced response is dose dependent and not necessarily restricted to an epidermis with Langerhans cells.

Studies in mice show the early phase of ACD (ear swelling, in mice) to be induced by hapten-specific CD3–CD4–CD8–Thy1+ cells, which can stimulate mast cells and recruit antigen-non-specific MHC-restricted late-acting CD3+CD4+CD8– T cells. The latter are responsible for the eczematous reaction. In the early phase, neuropeptides such as substance P, calcitonin-gene related product and somatostatin are capable of increasing the inflammation independent of the cause of contact dermatitis. They increase plasma extravasation and local blood flow. Calcitonin-gene related product, in contrast to other neuropeptides, has also been shown to boost sensitization.[3,4]

Investigations in different models argue for an active involvement of keratinocytes and other APCs in the elicitation phase. They liberate proinflammatory cytokines which activate endothelial cells, attract leucocytes and upregulate adhesion and MHC molecules. Among others, IL-1β, TNF-α, monocyte chemotactic protein-1, IFN-inducible protein-10 and macrophage inflammatory protein-1α have been identified to be involved in the mediator cascade. Cutaneous neuropeptides including calcitonin-gene related product and α-melanocyte stimulating hormone exert significant downregulating effects. A similar function has been suggested for IL-4. The induction of T-helper 1 (Th1) or Th2 type cytokines in ACD depends on the antigen. However, there is a tendency for IL-4 dominated Th2 responses in ACD and for Th1 responses (IFN-γ dominated) in other types of delayed-type hypersensitivity.

The role of expression of adhesion molecules is a crucial step in the early phase of ACD and blocking them on endothelial cells results in diminished responses. Their expression by epidermal keratinocytes seems to be a co-stimulatory event for an ongoing ACD.[1,2]

Immunologic differences between ACD and other types of delayed contact hypersensitivity are given in Table 2.2.

Irritant contact dermatitis

Haptens/antigens can cause not only ACD but also irritant reactions. It is assumed that haptens have a non-specific proinflammatory capacity that "conditions" skin for ACD and may induce irritant reactions as well. The primary cells involved in these early reactions are the epidermal keratinocytes, which is capable of liberating a variety of proinflammatory cytokines. Since their activation is not antigen specific a relatively high amount of hapten is necessary. The effect is dose dependent. The accumulation of leukocytes occurs after this first stimulus. If hapten-specific T cells are present in the infiltrate, they will become activated by hapten contact. This will lead to an amplification of inflammation, resulting in ACD.[2]

ICD has a far greater incidence than ACD and is characterized by non-specificity. Re-exposure to irritants can cause a breakdown of stratum corneum barrier function even at low doses. Higher doses may result in acute toxicity during first contact. As shown by electron resonance studies, anionic surfactants can bind to lipid membranes of the horny layer and increase the mobility of the bilayers. Higher mobility suggest a decrease in skin barrier function.[5] The breakdown of skin barrier function can improve hapten/antigen penetration into skin. ICD may therefore provide a basis for subsequent development of ACD. Interestingly, skin roughness is not related to ICD in humans[6] but dry skin is more prone to irritant reactions. The major target for irritant reactions is the epidermal keratinocytes, which can either be damaged or become activated, depending on the dose. The irritant interferes with metabolism and differentiation, leading to dyskeratosis and parakeratosis.[7] Activated keratinocytes liberate proinflammatory cytokines and provoke non-specific dose-dependent leucocyte attraction.[8] The upregulation of certain adhesion molecules such as $\alpha 6$ integrin or CD36 is independent of the stimulus (e.g. antigen or irritant) and is not cytokine induced. It has been related to the proliferative activity of keratinocytes.[9,10] Other adhesion molecules are activated by proinflammatory stimuli.

Though keratinocytes become activated and secrete proinflammatory cytokines, the Langerhans cells do not change their functional state as much as they do in ACD. Irritants do not have the capacity to induce IL-1β in Langerhans cells, which is essential for their migration into the lymph nodes.

References

1. Enk AH, Allergic contact dermatitis: understanding the immune response and potential for targeted therapy using cytokines. *Mol Med Today* 1997; **3**:423–438.

2. Grabbe S, Schwarz T, Immunoregulatory mechanisms involved in elicitation of allergic contact hypersensitivity. *Immunol Today* 1998; **19**:37–44.

3. Gutwald J, Goebeler M, Sorg C, Neuropeptides enhance irritant and allergic contact dermatitis. *J Invest Dermatol* 1991; **96**:695–698.

4. Wollina U, Gebhardt M, Lange D, Neuropeptide beim atopischen Ekzem und anderen Dermatosen. In: Garbe C, Rassner G (eds). *Dermatologie – Leitlinien und Qualitätssicherung für Diagnostik und Therapie.* Berlin: Springer; 1998:46–49.

5. Kawasaki Y, Quan D, Sakamoto K, Maibach HI, Electron resonance studies on the influence of anionic surfactants on human skin. *Dermatology* 1997; **194**:238–242.

6. Iliev D, Hinnen U, Elsner P, Skin roughness is negatively correlated to irritation with DMSO, but not with NaOH and SLS. *Exp Dermatol* 1997; **6**:157–160.

7. Willis CM, Stephens CJ, Wilkinson JD, Epidermal damage induced by irritants in man: a light and electron microscopic study. *J Invest Dermatol* 1989; **93**:695–699.

8. Nickoloff BJ, Naidu Y, Perturbation of epidermal barrier function correlates with initiation of cytokine cascade in human skin. *J Am Acad Dermatol* 1994; **30**:535–546.

9. Jung K, Imhof BA, Linse R, Wollina U, Neumann C, Adhesion molecules in atopic dermatitis: upregulation of α6 integrin expression in spontaneous lesional skin as well as in atopen, antigen and irritative induced patch test reactions. *Int Arch Allergy Immunol* 1997; **113**:495–504.

10. Willis CM, Stephens CJ, Wilkinson JD, Selective expression of immune-associated surface antigens by keratinocytes in irritant contact dermatitis. *J Invest Dermatol* 1991; **96**:505–511.

3. Basics of Patch Testing

Matthias Gebhardt

The diagnosis and evaluation of allergic contact dermatitis (ACD) are mainly made by carefully recording the patient's case history. Table 3.1 lists the items that should be considered when taking a patient's contact allergy history. The appearance of the skin rash (regional distribution), the time between exposure and first complaint, and the history of previous allergic reactions (chemical similarity between previous individual allergens and current contact substances) sometimes indicates a particular exposure situation. If such exposure is possibly allergenic in nature, then a "patch test" might be indicated to prove the hypothesis. It is important to save a sample of the suspected agent in the acute stage of the skin disease for patch tests later on.

To "patch test" is to apply a chemical or biological material to the intact, non-inflamed skin on the back of the individual who is suspected to have a contact allergy. This simple procedure was first introduced by Jadasson in 1896. He used cotton patches dampened with aqueous solutions of particular chemicals. Today, patch testing is made much more comfortable by using tapes, prefabricated with separate test chambers; these are available from several providers. A huge number of test substances is available, along with recommendations of test series for various professions, exposure situations, eczema patterns, etc. However, the interpretation of patch test results is as difficult as the procedure is simple. It requires excellent knowledge of possible exposure to different substances in the occupational environment, the composition of cosmetics and topical drugs, and botanical substances, and not least a rather "forensic" mind. Many technologies are changing rapidly, therefore it is always important to make sure that a type of exposure which has been generally well-known is still valid for the individual case; for example, flour bleaching has not been done with benzoyl peroxide for about four decades, paraphenylenediamine is no longer used for hair dyes in Europe, and cadmium pigments for manufacture of acrylic dentures were banned long ago.

When should a patch test be done?

A diagnostic patch test should be considered whenever an eczematous reaction has recently occurred for the first time in an adult. Although atopic dermatitis (AD) is a genetically based skin disease, some environmental factors may aggravate its course and, therefore, patch testing can sometimes help to identify triggering mechanisms. It may be the case that recalcitrant courses of almost any

Table 3.1 Case history and examination of contact allergy patients

Aspects to ask about when seeing a patient with suspected contact allergy	
Previous skin diseases	Individual history, family members affected
Onset of skin complaints	Age, location, repeating circumstances upon recurrence
Course	Self-limiting, relapsing or chronic
Symptoms	Itching, burning
Occupation	Current/previous vocational training
Leisure-time activities	Sports, gardening, plants, home building projects
Improvement	At weekends, when not at home, on vacation
Worsening	Upon sun exposure
Previous findings	Allergy history
Earlier intolerances	Fashion jewellery, cosmetics, textiles, rubber gloves, plants
Current medical treatment	New treatment, changes following seeing a doctor/dentist
Items to look for when seeing a patient with suspected contact allergy	
Distribution of clues to exposure	Hands involved? If yes, which part of hands (dorsal, palms, web spaces, finger sides)?
	Face: eyelids, perioral, lips
	Perianogenital
	Close to leg ulcer
	Skin folds (systemic contact dermatitis)
	Dorsal hands and face: restricted to sun-exposed areas?
Morphe	Epidermal involvement? papules, vesicles, erosions, scales, hyperkeratosis, rhagades
	Mucosal involvement: lichenoid, erythematous
Items to look for in differential diagnosis of contact dermatitis	
Areas typical for other dermatoses	Psoriasis: scalp, elbows, sacral region, finger and toe nails
	Seborrhoic eczema: retroauricular, eyelids, eyebrows, paranasal fold, sternal area
	Atopic dermatitis: flexural areas, neck, palms, etc.
Clinical signs	Atopy criteria: orbital darkening, Dennie–Morgan fold, keratosis pilaris, hyperlinear palms, white dermographism, etc.
	Psoriasis criteria: dandruff, anal rhagades

skin disease, particularly eczematous disease, can be illuminated by finding out aggravating contact allergens. Patch testing is also useful in the investigation for causative drugs in earlier drug rashes.

So-called prophetic patch testing is sometimes requested if an estimation of health risks with no previous but expected future contact with substances is required. This can be especially important in pre-employment screenings. However, if pre-employment history is not suggestive of antecedent contact allergy, pre-employment patch testing is unnecessary and usually leads to confusion and misinterpretation.[1] There are a few circumstances under which prophetic patch testing makes sense. It is probably only justified in challenging the individual with a new substance that crossreacts with another agent that previously lead to allergy.

What should be considered when doing patch tests?

Neither the skin of the back nor remote sites of the skin should be inflamed before patch testing because this would yield a state of increased irritability and false-positive reactions. Optimally, the patches are applied to the upper part of the back which is not overlying the spine. An alternative site for patch tests is the deltoid region of the upper arm. The skin should not be treated by any immunosuppressive agent such as UV, corticosteroids or other active agents. In patients suspected of having a fixed drug eruption, it is recommended that patch tests are done in the area of the eruption after resolution.

When testing products used by patients, one has to make sure that no strong irritant (tensides, acids, alkalines) is applied in an undiluted manner. Conversely, overdilution bears the risk of missing a test reaction because of below-threshold concentrations of the possible allergen. In rinse-off cosmetics for hair and body cleansing for example, irritant effects of tensides require dilutions down to 1%, at which level the preservative concentrations would be below the elicitation threshold. Substances that should not be tested in the form of complete product include strong alkaline bath and kitchen cleansers, construction materials, unknown plastic monomers, some flower and plant parts, glues etc. In these cases it is always better to test for individual ingredients (as far as they are declared). Patch testing of unknown products without labelled declaration of ingredients should not be done in routine practice (if ever).

Suboptimal patch test procedures or omitted precautions may lead to false-positive or false-negative reactions.

Most patch test materials are diluted in petrolatum or water, depending on solubility. Test chambers are round or square and made from aluminum or polyethylene plastic. Some allergens such as mercury compounds may be problematic when tested in aluminum test chambers, but in daily practice and except for scientific studies this is of limited importance. The easiest test device to use is the TRUE test (thin-layer rapid use epicutaneous test). This standardized ready-to-apply patch test system is made from polyester covered with a film of allergens incorporated in a hydrophilic polymer. The patches are mounted on non-woven cellulose tape with acrylic adhesive, covered with siliconized plastic and packed in an airtight and light-impermeable envelope. When the test strip is taped on the skin, perspiration hydrates the film and transforms it to a gel, which causes the allergen to be released.[2] There are, however, only two test panels each with 12 allergens available, which represent the full standard panel approved by government (FDA) for use in the USA.

There are some variations to the patch test such as those gien in Table 3.2.

Table 3.2 Variations to the patch test

Test	*Comments*
Open test	Optimal test for products used by patients' or substances of uncertain irritancy
Tape stripping	Common pre-treatment for testing eye drops, aeroallergens to enhance the absorption into the skin
24 or 48h application	Always controversial because 24h (vs. 48h) will miss some weak positive reactions whereas 48h (vs. 24h) is more likely to cause false-positive irritant reactions
Repeated open application test (ROAT)	Application of test material twice daily on the forearm for 2 weeks

Causes of false-positive and false-negative test reactions

False-positive results

- Angry back syndrome (syn. excited skin syndrome; strong test reactions adjacent to the false-positive reaction)
- Irritation by excess concentrations of the allergen or by the vehicle
- Active regional or remote skin disease

False-negative results

- Testing the wrong allergens (probably the most frequent cause)
- Allergen concentrations too low
- Local immunosuppression:
  - UV induced
  - after treatment with immunosuppressive topicals

- Systemic immunosuppression:
  - disease induced
  - drug induced
- Absence of co-factors such as UV light in photoallergic reactions
- Early detachment of the patch
- Stopping patch test reading too early

The last point is of special attention because some allergens, such as acrylates, corticosteroids, Compositae, neomycin and ethylene diamine, require delayed readings because otherwise one would miss a possible late reaction. It is very important to perform patch test readings after 48h, and optimally up to 96h. There is a particular need to do so if the patient is tested for medicolegal reasons. I perform routine readings after 1 week for acrylates, corticosteroids and Compositae. Neomycin is another substance for which results appear late. The importance of late readings was proven by Uter et al.[3] in a German multicentre study: 34.5% of all positive reactions appeared at day 3 only, whereas 8.3% of reactions initially judged (weakly) positive were not considered allergic at day 3.[3]

The evaluation of a test reaction: "relevance"

The biggest challenge for the dermatologist is deciding the nature of a positive reaction. Test reactions are rated positive (Figure 3.1) according to the International Contact Dermatitis Group (ICDRG) recommendation (Table 3.3).

When the morphology indicates a positive reaction, one has to decide whether it is allergic or irritant in nature. Irritant reactions are characterized by a decrescendo type of reaction, i.e. the reaction fades between the first and following readings, whereas crescendo or maintained positivity is more likely in allergic

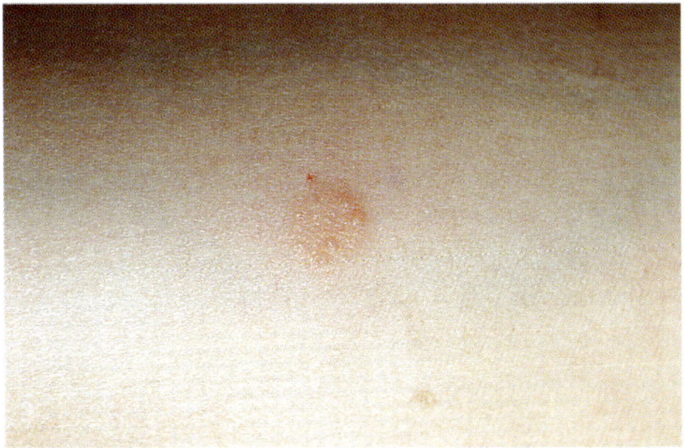

Figure 3.1: Positive patch test reaction (++).

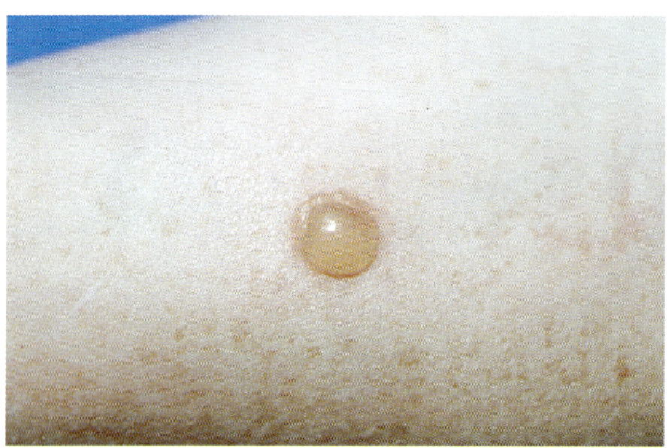

Figure 3.2: Bullous patch test reaction.

Table 3.3 Patch test reactions according to the ICDRG criteria

Reaction	*Description*	*May even contain:*
(+) or ?	Erythema without infiltration	
+	Infiltrated erythema	Discrete papules
++	Infiltrated erythema with papules	Discrete vesicles
+++	Infiltrated erythema with papules and coalescing vesicles	

reactions. Non-infiltrated homogeneous erythema, fine wrinkled surfaces in the test area, petechiae, pustules, blisters (Figure 3.2) and, finally, necrosis are other non-allergic features of a test reaction. Follicular papules without infiltrated erythema are possible in both irritant and allergic reactions. This type of reaction is especially common with metal salts. One can try to avoid patch test irritation by intradermal testing of type IV allergens with readings in the same time course; however, this principle has not found broad acceptance. Although morphological criteria have been defined, most allergists use their knowledge about the chemical substance in their test evaluation. Therefore, even slightly infiltrated erythematous reactions to highly reactive agents (e.g. benzoyl peroxide), emulgators (propylene glycol), fragrances or surface-active compounds (cocamidopropylbetaine, gallates, etc.) are preferentially rated as irritant reactions. This rating is closely associated with "relevance" estimation. Exposure lists of allergens are helpful to the patient in determining the "relevance" of a reaction and avoiding the allergen in the future. If the patient is exposed to allergen and the patient's dermatitis is explainable with regard to this exposure, then a test reaction can be referred to as relevant.[4] A patient may experience a genuine positive allergic reaction with different statements about relevance (Table 3.4).

Table 3.4 Relevance of a positive reaction

Relevant . . .	*Example*
. . . For current skin disease	Neomycin sensitization in a patient presenting with contact dermatitis surrounding a leg ulcer that has been treated with a neomycin-containing ointment
. . . For any previous skin disease	Nickel sensitization 20 years ago on the earlobes of the same patient
. . . As cross allergen	Gentamicin sensitization in the same patient, without any preceding contact to this substance
No relevance	Reaction to chromates with no former suspicion of chromate-induced contact dermatitis

The concept of relevance is so important because many test reactions with typical morphological features of positivity (papules, erythema, infiltration) may bear no relation to any current or previous allergic condition. It would not help the patient to get information about such an allergen. Of course, the dermatologist should try very hard to prove the relevance of a test reaction; any 'non-relevant' statement may be false because necessary information has not been asked for or has been ignored. Non-relevant positive test reactions are not uncommon for mercury compounds.

Because of the tremendous importance of any statement about relevance, the patch test reaction should be thoroughly discussed with the patient after the final reading (Figures 3.1 and 3.2). If more information is required to obtain a relevance statement, the manufacturer of the products should be asked or chemical analysis should be considered.[5] Chemical analysis is not usually practicable in a doctor's office, but in university departments it should always be considered. Some easy-to-use chemical assays are commercially available for detecting formaldehyde in liquids (Merck formaldehyde test strips) and nickel release from metal alloys (dimethyl glyoxime test, from several providers).

Cross sensitization

Cross allergy is a sensitization to a chemical structure that can occur in various substances. An example is *para*-group allergy. Individuals reacting to paraphenylenediamine are likely to react to other chemicals that have related structures, such as azo dyes, sulphonamides and local anaesthetics. The same is true for antibiotics (gentamicin, neomycin, kanamycin and framycetin), corticosteroids, acrylates and many other groups of allergens. Some allergens seem to cross react but do not contain the same structures. This may be due to concomitant occurrence in the environment or in the test preparation. Balsam of Peru, for example, contains several fragrances that are also components of the fragrance mix test preparation, e.g. cinnamic aldehyde, cinnamic alcohol, eugenol and isoeugenol. Different metals occur together in particular alloys; this may be one reason why palladium as well as cobalt sensitization are almost always combined with nickel sensititization.

Compound allergy

This describes a test reaction to the compound *mixture* but not to all the individual ingredients when they are tested separately. An overview is given by Bashir and Maibach.[6] Five requirements are given to fulfil the criteria of compound allergy:

- The reaction must be allergic and not irritant
- The patch test for the constituents of the preparation must be negative
- The whole preparation must give a positive reaction on patch testing
- All the ingredients must be known and tested
- Vehicle-dependent contact allergy must be excluded

An irritant reaction may explain this phenomenon, as may the formation of a new allergen by mixing the components. The difference between the original vehicle(s) and the patch test vehicle has also been given as an explanation.

Connubial dermatitis

This term describes a contact reaction occurring not only in the exposed individual but also in their contacts (e.g. spouses). Fragrances, cosmetics and topical drugs are typical causes of connubial dermatitis. Although the cause seems quite simple to identify, it may be difficult to determine relevant exposure.

Proofs of relevance

In view of the artificiality of occluded tape application, there is no doubt that more genuine tests are required. The "use test", in the form of ROAT, has been considered proof of relevance by many authors. The patch test substance or the consumer product should be applied twice daily for 14 days on the volar aspect of the forearm or on the cubital area. As soon as an eczematous reaction occurs, the test is stopped. However, there are variations in the outcome in patch-test positive patients, with false-positive irritant reactions. Use of two test preparations, first the allergen incorporated into a vehicle, and second the vehicle itself, may improve the results because irritancy due to the vehicle can be excluded.

Workplace-related exposure may be mimicked by asking the individual to do some aspect of her or his particular job. So, the baker may knead dough, the florist make a bunch of flowers, etc., in the dermatologists office. Flare up of the eczematous condition during a period of what is otherwise activity restriction (sick leave, vacation, etc.) can be attributed to such a realistic challenge procedure. If the antecedent eczema location flares during patch testing, that would be an indicator that a given test reaction is relevant.

Another proof of relevance can be oral provocation. Some allergens have been given orally for diagnostic purposes in type IV allergy, such as nickel, balsam of Peru and drug substances, others have yielded flares when taken by mistake (antabuse in thiuram allergics, flavours and spices in fragrance allergics, etc.).

Risks of patch testing

There are some health hazards associated with patch tests, although the test procedure is generally safe. The major serious problems are active sensitization and

Table 3.5 Risks associated with patch test

Problem	*Prognosis*
Active sensitization	Remaining state of the immune system
Booster of weak sensitization	Remaining state of the immune system
Anaphylactic reactions upon epicutaneous re-exposure	Serious condition with critical outcome
Flare of previous eczema sites	Slowly fading condition
Long-lasting test reactions	Slowly fading test site reaction
Pigmentation of skin	Slowly fading test site reaction
Pigmentation of clothing	Remaining/partly remaining
False-positive test reaction with misleading conclusions	Depending on situation
False-negative test reaction with missing elicitor	Depending on situation

severe anaphylactoid reactions upon re-exposure to a given substance. The former is likely to occur when a patch test reaction appears late, after a week or later. The latter is rarely a problem with standard patch test substances but can occur with medicaments, enzymes or proteins, e.g. latex. Table 3.5 lists some more points to be taken into consideration when making conclusions from patch tests.

Any patch test should be done only after avoidable risk factors have been excluded. This is the reason why patch testing should be avoided in pregnant women, although serious significant risks are unlikely. People who want to be patch tested for exclusion or ask for repeated proof of allergy are at risk of being actively sensitized, too. This is the case with dental materials in patients who fear amalgam or burning mouth syndrome. It is the responsibility of the allergist or dermatologist not to apply a patch test without reasonable indication. A previously obtained positive test result should not be reproduced, if relevance has already been ascertained. Any positive reaction increases the reactivity of the surrounding skin: so retesting known allergens increases the risk of obtaining too many false-positive results. Patch testing is also deceptive when the person who performs the test is uncritical in relying on the test results and draws wrong conclusions from false-positive or false-negative results.

It is important to recognize that patch test reproducibility is all but 100%. The test can only be an auxiliary procedure in contact allergy diagnosis. Knowledge of exposure and the patient's history and understanding of the chemistry is essential to make a good diagnosis on the basis of this artificial assay.

Influences on patch test epidemiology

Patch test results are influenced by many factors but mainly by sex and age. When looking at trends in contact dermatitis development, these population-based factors have to be taken into consideration. The MOAHL index has been chosen to give a standardization factor for certain populations in epidemiological studies of contact allergy: (M = male, O = occupational dermatitis, A = age, H = hand eczema, L = leg ulcer). Facial dermatitis and age above 40 years has been proposed by Schnuch et al. for an extended index.[7]

It is worth looking at two examples of the role of those population-based factors. First, it is known that nickel allergy is much more common among young women than among males or elderly women. Therefore, any change in the rate of nickel allergy should be checked for concomitant changes in age or sex profiles of the examined group; regional differences should also be discussed. Thimerosal sensitization is much more prevalent in regions with a higher rate of vaccinations, such as FSME (tick-borne encephalitis) endemic regions; this phenomenon has been observed in the middle European region where a tremendous increase of thimerosal sensitization is seen from North Germany to Austria.

Summary

The patch test is a complex model of and diagnostic tool for ACD. Compared with other diagnostic procedures it is not particularly harmful. Factors that contribute to reliable diagnosis of ACD are a well-recorded case history, the choice of appropriate patch test substances and concentrations, careful patch test reading and a well-founded relevance statement. Patch test results are more reliable for eczematous disorders than for eczematous conditions but not that reliable for non-eczematous conditions such as drug rashes, urticarial disorders or mucosal symptoms.

References

1. Mathias CGT, Prevention of occupational contact dermatitis. *J Am Acad Dermatol* 1990; **23:**742–748.

2. Fischer T, Maibach HI, Easier patch testing with TRUE Test. *J Am Acad Dermatol* 1989 **20:**447–453.

3. Uter WJ, Geier J, Schnuch A, Good clinical practice in patch testing: readings beyond day 2 are necessary: a confirmatory analysis. Members of the Information Network of Departments of Dermatology. *Am J Contact Dermat* 1996; **7:**231–237.

4. Wilkinson DS, Fregert S, Magnusson B et al, Terminology of contact dermatitis. *Acta Derm Venereol (Stockh)* 1970; **50:**287–292.

5. Ale SI, Maibach HI, Clinical relevance in allergic contact dermatitis. *Dermatosen* 1995; **43:**119–121.

6. Bashir SJ, Maibach HI, Compound allergy. *Contact Dermatitis* 1997; **36:**179–83.

7. Schnuch A, Geier J, Uter W et al, National rates and regional differences in sensitisation to allergens of the standard series – population-adjusted frequencies of sensitisation (PAFS) in 40,000 patients from a multicenter study (IVDK). *Contact Dermatitis* 1997; **37:**200–209.

4. Irritant Contact Dermatitis

Dimiter Iliev and Peter Elsner

Introduction

Irritant contact dermatitis (ICD) is an important and often underestimated problem in dermatology.[1,2] ICD is probably more frequent than allergic contact dermatitis (ACD), although reliable data are still very limited. In contrast to other groups of diseases it is not a clinical entity but rather a spectrum of diseases and in contrast to ACD, ICD is defined as being the result of primarily non-specific damage to the skin (Table 4.1). The clinical picture of ICD is determined by a dose–effect relationship.[3] ICD can occur in any individual, provided that irritants are in contact with the skin for a sufficient length of time and are in sufficiently high concentration.

Most frequently affected by ICD are the hands, because they are the human "tools" that interact with the environment most and have intensive contact with irritants. However, spilling of fluids may irritate the forearms or other body sites, especially when fluids soak through work clothes. The incidence of irritant dermatitis correlates with the exposure of workers in a given profession.[4] Some high-risk occupations are: caterers,[5] furniture industry workers,[6] hospital workers[7] (nurses,[8] cleaners,[9] kitchen workers), hairdressers,[10] chemical industry workers,[11] dry cleaners,[12] metal workers,[13–16] florists[17] and warehouse workers.[18] Airborne irritant dermatitis develops in irritant-exposed sensitive skin, mostly the face and especially the periorbital region.[19,20] Irritant dermatitis caused by dust may mimic textile dermatitis, with lesions most prominent in sites of close skin–garment contact, e.g. the axilla, gluteal region and thighs.

The morphology of ICD includes erythema, oedema, vesicles that may coalesce, bullae and oozing. Necrosis is only seen with primary irritants. The

Table 4.1 Irritant versus allergic contact dermatitis

	ICD	*ACD*
Diseased skin	All exposed areas	Only sensitized areas
Concentration dependency	Dose effect	"All or nothing"
Subjective qualities	Burning, stinging	Itching
Objective qualities	Erythema, oedema, bulla, necrosis, desquamation	Erythema, papule, vesicle
Diagnosis	No diagnostic test	Patch test

clinical features of chronic ICD include redness, lichenification, excoriations, scaling and hyperkeratosis. Several types of ICD have been described. However, the pathophysiologic process should always be considered to be of multi-step–multiethiologic origin. ICD can be regarded as a diagnosis of exclusion, in which no allergic cause is detected.

When assessing the acute or cumulative irritancy of products it is mostly limited to weak or diluted irritants. Either patch or "use" tests can be performed. Increased sensitivity and quantification of the irritants can be achieved by a bioengineering assessment. Applying non-invasive bioengineering methods it is possible to target the irritant, the irritated or the irritation. In recent years, these methods have been increasingly applied in the physiological and patho-physiological characterization of human skin in vivo. Thus the idea of applying different bioengineering methods seems to be a good approach in order to quantify the different symptoms of ICD in terms of intensity and quality.

Another important approach is to quantify the individual features of humans which make them susceptible to ICD by measuring their irritant resistance. This suggestion was made by Burckhard in 1935[21] who designed the alkali resistance test. Newer irritants include sodium lauryl sulphate (SLS) and dimethyl sulphox-ide (DMSO).

Despite their different pathogenesis, ACD and ICD, especially in their chronic forms, show a remarkable similarity with respect to clinical appearance, histology,[22,23] and immunohistology.[24,25] Frequently, even their therapy is similar.[26,27] The histological pattern of chronic ICD is characterized by hyperkeratosis with areas of parakeratosis, moderate-to-marked acanthosis, elongation of the rete ridges and moderate mononuclear perivascular infiltrates.[28] Under both electron and light microscopy,[29] acute ICD histologically shows morphological damage in the epidermis.

Clinical types of ICD

Several different types of ICD have been described:[30,31]

- Acute
- Acute delayed
- Irritant reaction
- Cumulative
- Traumiterative
- Xerotic eczema (craquele)
- Traumatic
- Pustular and acneiform
- Non-erythematous
- Subjective or sensory

Acute ICD

Acute ICD, also called irritant reaction, develops when the skin is exposed to a potent irritant (Figure 4.1). Usually this happens as an accident at work or in special emergency situations. The irritant reaction reaches its peak quickly and then starts to heal. This is called the "decrescendo phenomenon". Because the lag time is short (usually minutes to hours after exposure) and the association between exposure and skin symptoms are usually clear, the diagnosis is easy in most cases. It may become difficult when the patient is unaware of any exposure. Acute ACD has to be considered as differential diagnosis, which is caused by a delayed sensitization reaction and requires 24–48h after allergen contact before symptoms appear. This type of contact dermatitis is characterized by the "crescendo phenomenon", i.e. a transient increase of signs and symptoms despite removal of the allergen. The clinical appearance of acute ICD is very variable, and it may even be indistinguishable from the allergic type. There are numerous reports in the literature of even experienced dermatologists being misled into an initial assumption of ACD which later, after a careful work-up, turns out to be "only irritation".[32] Furthermore, the combination of ACD and ICD is frequent, e.g. the black-spot poison ivy dermatitis described by Hurwitz et al.[33] as acute ICD superimposed upon ACD.

Symptoms of acute ICD are burning, stinging, and soreness of the skin. Signs are erythema, oedema, bullae and possibly necrosis. The lesions are restricted to

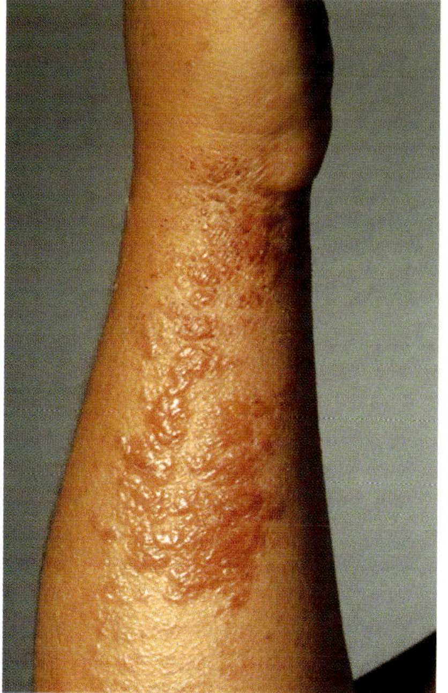

Figure 4.1: Irritant contact dermatitis of the forearm due to jellyfish.

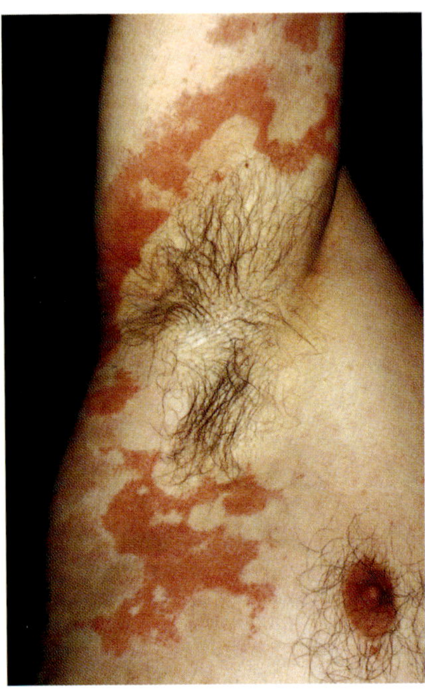

Figure 4.2: Acute irritant contact dermatitis.

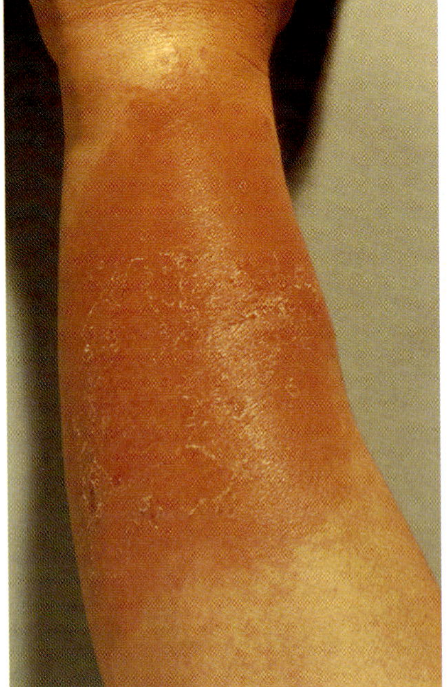

Figure 4.3: Acute irritant contact dermatitis of the forearm due to tear-gas.

the area where the irritant or toxicant damaged the tissue. Their borders are sharply demarcated, and their asymmetrical pattern hints at an exogenous cause. The prognosis of this type of ICD is good.[34]

The most frequent potent irritants leading to ICD are acids and alkaline solutions.[35] A typical accident situation is chemical burning in construction workers,[36] when alkaline concrete fluid soaks through garments or spills into work boots. Chemical burns by fluoric acid are the most dangerous of all injuries caused by acids and need special treatment. But even substances thought to be less toxic, such as *N*-methyl-2-pyrrolidone, may cause acute ICD (Figures 4.2 and 4.3).[37]

Acute delayed ICD

Acute delayed ICD is characteristic of certain irritants, such as anthralin, that elicit a retarded inflammatory response. Clinically, acute delayed ICD resembles acute ICD. The visible inflammation is not seen until 8–24 h or more after exposure.[38] Delayed irritation may be more common than generally thought so far. Other substances causing it include benzalkonium chloride and tretinoin. Irritant patch test reactions to benzalkonium chloride may be papular and increase in intensity with time, thus imitating ACD. On the normal skin surrounding psoriatic plaques, dithranol causes redness and oedema, which may become very severe on the legs due to venous stasis. Irritation due to tretinoin develops after a few days and is characterized by mild to fiery redness, followed by desquamation of large flakes of stratum corneum. The symptoms are burning rather than itching. The skin becomes sensitive to touch and to water (Figure 4.4).[32]

Irritant reaction ICD

Irritant reaction ICD is a type of subclinical irritant dermatitis in individuals exposed to liquids, such as hairdressers or metal workers in their first months of training. This diagnosis is made if the clinical picture is monomorphic rather than polymorphic and characterized by one or more of the following signs: scaling, redness, vesicles, pustules and erosions.[32]

On the hands it often begins under rings and then may spread over the fingers to the hands and the forearms. It usually affects the dorsum of the hands and fingers, but irritants can also cause eczema of the palmar sides of the fingers and hands. This distribution occurs in caterers and, described as dyshidrotic eczema, it has been reported in metal workers with ICD due to cooling lubricants.[5] Frequently, this condition heals spontaneously, resulting in hardening of the skin; sometimes it progresses to cumulative irritant dermatitis.

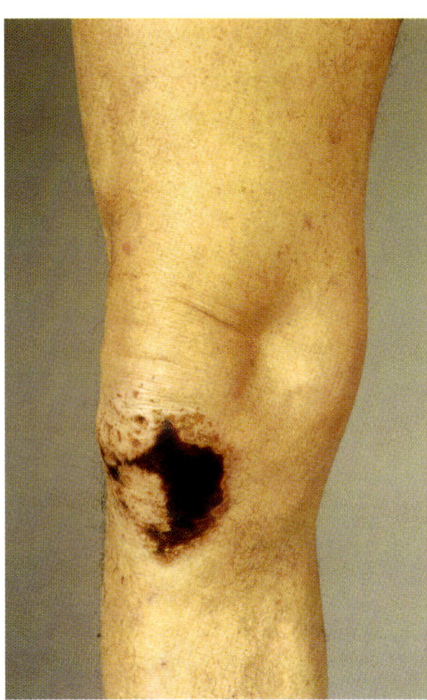

Figure 4.4: Irritant contact dermatitis due to cement.

Cumulative ICD

In contrast to acute ICD, cumulative ICD is a consequence of multiple subthreshold damage to the skin, in which the time between the insults is too short for complete restoration of skin barrier function. It may be the result of too frequent repetition of one impairing factor, but is more commonly the result of a variety of stimuli, each becoming active before recovery from the earlier stimuli has been completed. Clinical symptoms will develop only when the damage exceeds a certain "manifestation threshold", which is individually determined. People with "sensitive skin" are characterized by a decreased threshold and/or an increased restoration time, leading to earlier development of clinical irritant dermatitis. The threshold is not a fixed value for an individual, but it may decrease with the disease. This explains why for patients with cumulative ICD even limited irritant exposure may perpetuate the condition.

Cumulative ICD is linked not to exposure to a potent irritant, but to exposure to weak irritants. Very often, this exposure occurs not only at work but also in private life. Because the link between exposure and disease is often not obvious to the patient, diagnosis may be delayed considerably. This is one of the reasons for the rather doubtful prognosis of the disease.[39]

Symptoms of chronic irritant dermatitis are itching and pain due to cracking of hyperkeratotic skin. Signs include dryness, erythema and vesicles, but the

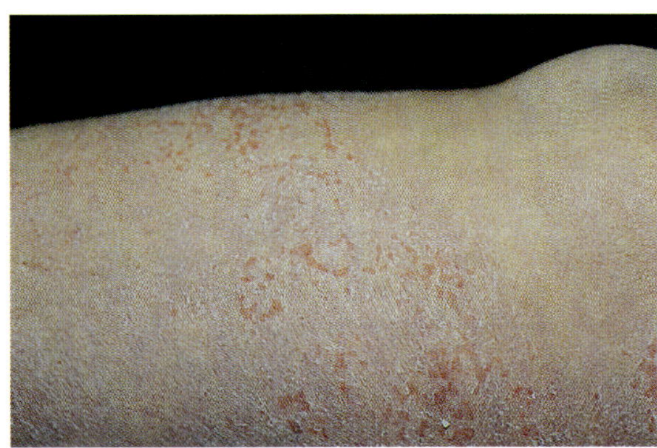

Figure 4.5: Exsiccation eczematid (eczema craquelé).

main signs are lichenification, hyperkeratosis, and chapping. In contrast to acute irritant dermatitis, the lesions are less sharply demarcated. Xerotic dermatitis is the most frequent type of cumulative toxic dermatitis.[35]

Many bioassays have been proposed for the purpose of identifying sensitive skin. A 24h patch test with SLS and repetitive patch test, such as the 21-day cumulative irritation assay, the chamber scarification test, and the soap chamber test have been used.[40]

Traumiterative ICD

While cumulative ICD results from repetition of exposure that differ in type, traumiterative ICD is a result of repetition of just one type of load.[29] Nevertheless these two types are very similar clinically.

Xerotic ecze,a (craquele)

Exsiccation eczematid (Figure 4.5) is a special variant of ICD that is seen mainly in elderly individuals with a history of frequent showering and/or bathing without remoisturizing their skin. Patients suffer from intensive itching, and their skin appears dry with ichthyosiform scaling. The condition mainly occurs during the winter months when humidity is low.

Traumatic ICD

This may develop after acute skin trauma like burns, lacerations and acute ICD. Patients should also be asked whether they have cleansed the skin with strong soaps or detergents. The syndrome is characterized by eczematous lesions and delayed healing. This eczematous condition persists for a considerable time period, with a minimum of 6 weeks.[32] The most common location is the hands. In a fully developed case redness, infiltration and scaling with fissuring is seen all over the affected areas.

Pustular and acneiform ICD

This is a result of exposure to certain irritants such as croton oil, mineral oils, tars, greases and naphthalenes. This syndrome has always to be considered in conditions in which acneiform lesions develop outside the typical acne age range. The people most affected are patients with seborrhoea, macroporous skin conditions or former acne vulgaris, as well as atopics. The pustules are sterile and transient. However, subcorneal pustular eruption may also be a manifestation of allergy to trichlorethylene, which has to be considered as a differential diagnosis in patients who have an appropriate history.[41]

Non-erythematous ICD

This may be defined as a subclinical form of ICD with early stages of skin irritation characterized only by changes in the stratum corneum barrier function without a clinical correlate.

Subjective or sensory ICD

This is characterized by its lack of clinical signs. Sick individuals report a stinging or burning feeling after contact with certain chemicals such as lactic acid, which is also a model irritant for this type of non-visible cutaneous irritation. This reaction may be reliably reproduced in a double-blind exposure test. Important parameters are the quality and the concentration of the exposing agent. Neural pathways are considered to be responsible.[31]

Summary

Clinical manifestations of the ICD syndromes are modified by external factors (type of irritant, exposure, and environmental factors such as mechanical pressure, temperature and humidity) and depend on predisposing characteristics of the individual[42] (age, sex, ethnic origin, pre-existing skin disease, especially atopic skin diathesis, and anatomical region exposed[43]). For instance, older people are not only affected more often by contact dermatitis because of their lower epidermal barrier but show also more severe symptoms of this disease.[44,45] Environmental influences such as low ambient humidity and cold are important factors in decreasing the water content of the stratum corneum.[46] Cold alone may also reduce the plasticity of the horny layer, with consequent cracking of the stratum corneum. Occlusion increases the water content of the stratum corneum, with consequent enhanced percutaneous absorption of water-soluble substances.

References

1. Elsner P, Wilhelm D , Maibach HI, Multiple parameter assessment of vulvar irritant contact dermatitis. *Contact Dermatitis* 1990; **1**:20–26.
2. Klaus MV, Wieselthier JS, Contact dermatitis. *Am Fam Physician* 1993; **4**:629–632.
3. Mai Le TK, Schalwijk J, van de Kerkhof PCM et al., A histological and immunohistological study on chronic irritant contact dermatitis. *Contact Dermatitis* 1988; **9**:23–28.
4. Goldner R, Work-related irritant contact dermatitis. *Occup Med* 1994; **1**:37–44.
5. Cronin E, Dermatitis of the hands in caterers. *Contact Dermatitis* 1987; **17**:265–269.
6. Gan SL, Goh CL, Lee CS, Occupational dermatitis among sanders in the furniture industry. *Contact Dermatitis* 1987; **17**:237–240.
7. Gawkrodger DJ, Lloyd MH, Hunter JA, Occupational skin disease in hospital cleaning and kitchen workers. *Contact Dermatitis* 1986; **15**:132–135.
8. Kassis V, Vedel P , Darre E, Contact dermatitis to methyl methacrylate. *Contact Dermatitis* 1984; **1**:26–28.
9. Singgih SI, Lantinga H, Nater JP, Occupational hand dermatoses in hospital cleaning personnel. *Contact Dermatitis* 1986; **14**:14–19.
10. van der Walle HB, Brunsveld VM, Dermatitis in hairdressers. (I). The experience of the past 4 years. *Contact Dermatitis* 1994; **4**:217–221.
11. Hogan DJ, Review of contact dermatitis for non-dermatologists. *J Fla Med Assoc* 1990; **7**:663–666.
12. Aoki T, Kageyama R, [Three cases of dry cleaning dermatitis.] *Nippon Hifuka Gakkai Zasshi* 1989; **9**:1035–1038.
13. de Boer EM, van Ketel WG , Bruynzeel DP, Dermatoses in metal workers. (II). Allergic contact dermatitis. *Contact Dermatitis* 1989; **4**:280–286.
14. de Boer EM, van Ketel WG, Bruynzeel DP, Dermatoses in metal workers. (I). Irritant contact dermatitis. *Contact Dermatitis* 1989; **3**:212–218.
15. Foulds IS, Koh D, Dermatitis from metalworking fluids. *Clin Exp Dermatol* 1990; **15**:157–162.

16. Goh CL, Yuen R, A study of occupational skin disease in the metal industry (1986–1990). *Ann Acad Med Singapore* 1994; **5**:639–644.

17. Bangha E , Elsner P, Occupational dermatitis towards sesquiterpene lactones in a florist. *Am J Contact Dermatitis* 1996; **7**:188–90.

18. Ashworth J, Rycroft RJ, Waddy RS, Irritant contact dermatitis in warehouse employees. *Occup Med* 1993; **43**:32–34.

19. Dooms-Goossens AE, Debuschere KM, Gevers DM, Contact dermatitis caused by airborne agents. A review and case reports. *J Am Acad Dermatol* 1986; **15**:1–10.

20. Lachapelle JM, Industrial airborne irritant or allergic contact dermatitis. *Contact Dermatitis* 1986; **14**:137–145.

21. Burckhard W, Die Rolle des Alkali in der Pathogenese des Ekzems speziell des Gewerbeekzems. *Archiv Dermatol Syphilis* 1995; **173**:155–167.

22. Brand CU, Hunziker T, Braathen LR, Studies on human skin lymph containing Langerhans cells from sodium lauryl sulphate contact dermatitis. *J Invest Dermatol* 1992; **5**:109s–110s.

23. Brand CU, Hunziker T, Limat A et al., Large increase of Langerhans cells in human skin lymph derived from irritant contact dermatitis. *Br J Dermatol* 1993; **2**:184–188.

24. Brasch J, Burgard J , Sterry W, Common pathogenetic pathways in allergic and irritant contact dermatitis. *J Invest Dermatol* 1992; **2**:166–170.

25. Marks JG Jr, Zaino RJ, Bressler MF et al., Changes in lymphocyte and Langerhans cell populations in allergic and irritant contact dermatitis. *Int J Dermatol* 1987; **6**:354–357.

26. Binnick AN, Allergic and irritant contact dermatitis.*Compr Ther* 1981; **1**:17–21.

27. Lauerma AI, Stein BD, Homey B et al., Topical FK506: suppression of allergic and irritant contact dermatitis in the guinea pig. *Arch Dermatol Res* 1994; **6**:337–340.

28. Lever WF, Schaumburg-Lever G, Histopathology of the skin. In: Cooke DB, Patterson D, Smith LD et al. *Noninfectious vesicular and bullous diseases.* Philadelphia: Lippincott; 1990:101–51.

29. Malten KE, den Arend JA, Irritant contact dermatitis. Traumiterative and cumulative impairment by cosmetics, climate, and other daily loads. *Derm Beruf Umwelt* 1985; **4**:125–132.

30. Berardesca E, Distante F, Mechanisms of skin irritation. In: Elsner P, Maibach HI, eds. *Irritant dermatitis. New clinical and experimental aspects.* Basel: Karger; 1995:1–8.

31. Lammintausta K, Maibach HI, Contact dermatitis due to irritation: general principles, etiology, and histology. In: Adams RM, ed. *Occupational skin disease*. Philadelphia: WB Saunders; 1990:1–15

32. Frosch PJ, Cutaneous irritation. In: Rycroft RJG ed. *Textbook of contact dermatitis*, Berlin: Springer; 1992: 28–61.

33. Hurwitz RM, Rivera HP, Guin JD, Black-spot poison ivy dermatitis. An acute irritant contact dermatitis superimposed upon an allergic contact dermatitis. *Am J Dermatopathol* 1984; **4**:319–322.

34. Elsner P, Irritant dermatitis in the workplace. *Dermatol Clin* 1994; **3**:461–467.

35. Eichmann A, Amgwerd D, Toxische Kontaktdermatitis. *Schweiz Rundsch Med Prax* 1992; **19**:615–617.

36. Skogstad M, Levy F, Occupational irritant contact dermatitis and fungal infection in construction workers. *Contact Dermatitis* 1994; **1**:28–30.

37. Leira HL, Tiltnes A, Svendsen K et al., Irritant cutaneous reactions to *N*-methyl-2-pyrrolidone (NMP). *Contact Dermatitis* 1992; **3**:148–150.

38. Malten KE, den Arend JA, Wiggers RE, Delayed irritation: hexanediol diacrylate and butanediol diacrylate. *Contact Dermatitis* 1979; **3**:178–184.

39. Elsner P, Maibach HI, Irritant and allergic contact dermatitis. In: Elsner P, Martius J, eds. *Vulvovaginitis*. New York: M Dekker; 1993: 61–82.

40. Lee CH, Maibach HI, Study of cumulative irritant contact dermatitis in man utilizing open application on subclinically irritated skin. *Contact Dermatitis* 1994; **5**:271–275.

41. Goh CL, Noneczematous contact reactions In: Rycroft RJG, ed. *Textbook of contact dermatitis*. Berlin: Springer; 1992: 221–236.

42. Pinnagoda J, Tupker RA, Smit JA et al., The intra- and inter-individual variability and reliability of transepidermal water loss measurements. *Contact Dermatitis* 1989; **4**:255–259.

43. Emtestam L, Ollmar S, Electrical impedance index in human skin: measurements after occlusion, in 5 anatomical regions and in mild irritant contact dermatitis. *Contact Dermatitis* 1993; **2**:104–108.

44. Ghadially R, Brown BE, Sequeira Martin SM et al., The aged epidermal permeability barrier. Structural, functional, and lipid biochemical abnormalities in humans and a senescent murine model. *J Clin Invest* 1995; **5**:2281–2290.

45. Patil S, Maibach HI, Effect of age and sex on the elicitation of irritant contact dermatitis. *Contact Dermatitis* 1994; **5**:257–264.

46. Mozzanica N, Pathogenetic aspects of allergic and irritant contact dermatitis. *Clin Dermatol* 1992; **2**:115–121.

5. Contact Urticaria and Protein Contact Dermatitis

Theodor Karamfilow

Contact urticaria is a transient, wheal-and-flare reaction that appears where certain agents contact the skin.[1] Lesions occur within minutes to an hour after the cutaneous contact, and they disappear within 24h or less. Some contactants affect normal (intact) skin whereas others require damaged (eczematized or fissured) skin to produce urticaria.[2,3] Contact urticaria may be produced by non-immunological or immunological (IgE-mediated) mechanisms.

Non-immunological contact urticaria

Non-immunological contact urticaria arises without previous sensitization in most exposed individuals, and it is the most common type. It is due to release of vasoactive substances without the involvement of immunological processes.[4] In contrast to immunologically mediated urticaria, the reaction remains localized and does not cause systemic symptoms or spread to become generalized urticaria. Typically, the strength of this type of contact urticaria reaction varies from erythema to an urticarial response, depending on the concentration, skin site and substance (Table 5.1). The exact mechanism of the non-immunological contact urticarial reactions is not known, but it is suggested to be a direct effect on dermal blood vessels or by the non-antibody-mediated release of inflammatory mediators such as histamine, prostaglandin, leukotriene and substance P (Figure 5.1).[4]

Immunological contact urticaria

Immunological contact urticaria is caused by an antigen–antibody, type I (according to Gell and Coombs), IgE-mediated hypersensitivity reaction. Elevated serum levels of specific IgE antibodies to contact urticariogens such as natural latex have been demonstrated in association with immunological contact urticaria. The antigen (contact urticant) penetrates through the epidermis and reacts with specific IgE antibodies on the surface of dermal mast cells. This triggers degranulation and liberation of vasoactive substances, mainly histamine. Histamine and other mediators of inflammation (e.g. prostaglandin, leukotriene, kinin) may influence the degree of cutaneous symptoms, erythema and oedema.

Table 5.1 Agents producing non-immunological contact urticaria

Animals	*Fragrances and flavourings*
Arthropods	Balsam of Peru
Caterpillars	Benzaldehyde
Corals	Cassia (cinnamon oil)
Jellyfish	Cinnamic acid
Moths	Cinnamic aldehyde
Sea anemones	
	Metals
Foods	Cobalt
Cayenne pepper	
Fish	*Plant products*
Thyme	Nettles
	Seaweed
Medicaments	
Alcohols	*Preservatives*
Benzocaine	Benzoic acid
Camphor	Formaldehyde
Cantharides	Sodium benzoate
Capsaicin	Sorbic acid
Chloroform	
Dimethyl sulphoxide	*Miscellaneous*
Friar's balsam	Butyric acid
Methyl salicylate	Diethyl fumarate
Mustard (black)	Pine oil
Myrrh	Turpentine
Nicotinic acid esters	
Resorcinol	
Tar extracts	
Tincture of benzoin	
Witch hazel	

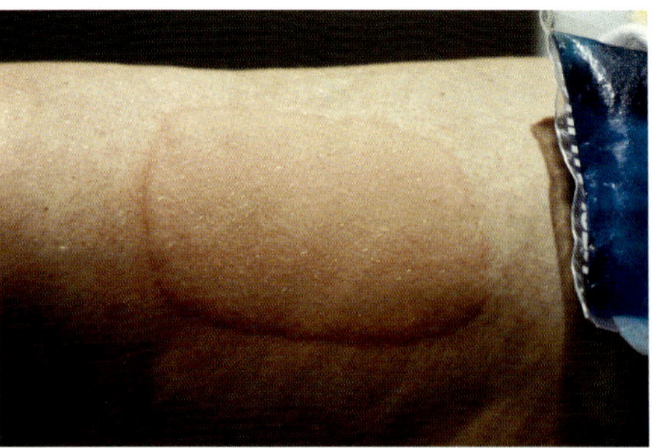

Figure 5.1: Physically induced urticaria due to cold.

Skin symptoms may be accompanied by other symptoms, such as rhinitis, conjunctivitis, asthma and anaphylactic shock.

Contact urticaria may be caused by other immunological mechanisms not requiring IgE antibodies; specific IgG or IgM antibodies might be responsible by activation of the complement cascade through the classic pathway.[3,5] Medications, foods, animal and plant products, metals and cosmetic ingredients can produce contact urticaria (Table 5.2).

The clinical presentation of contact urticaria comprises a spectrum from localized cutaneous reactions to involvement of extracutaneous organs. Maibach

Table 5.2 Selected agents that have been reported to produce contact urticaria

Medicaments	*Foods*
Bacitracin	Apple
Cephalosporin	Potato
Chloramphenicol	Bean
Gentamycin	Caraway seed
Neomycin	Carrot
Penicillin G	Egg
Streptomycin	Endive
Cephalosporins	Fish
Acetylsalicylic acid	Flour
Cetyl and stearyl alcohol	Lettuce
Estrogenic cream	Chicken
Tetanus antitoxin	Beer
Menthol	Lamb
Benzophenone	Beef
Mechlorethamine hydrochloride	Pork
Chlorpromazine	Milk
Polyethylene glycol	Peach
Polysorbate 60	Spices
Others	*Cosmetics*
Seminal fluid	Hair sprays
Pollens	Nail polish
Rubber	Perfumes
Animals	*Industrial exposure*
Animal hair	Platinum salts
Dog and cat saliva	Acrylic monomer
Animal dander	Lindane
Cow placenta	Aliphatic polyamide
Cockroaches	Aminothyazole
	Sodium sulphide

and Johnson[6] called this spectrum the "contact urticarial syndrome" and divided it into four stages:

- Stage 1: localized urticaria restricted to the area of contact
- Stage 2: generalized urticaria including angioedema
- Stage 3: urticaria associated with bronchial asthma
- Stage 4: urticaria associated with anaphylactoid reactions.

The diagnosis of contact urticaria is essentially based on a carefully taken history. In vivo skin testing with suspected agents and in vitro testing with the radioallergosorbent test (RAST) completes the diagnostic process. Skin testing for contact urticaria should be monitored carefully to control potentially life-threatening anaphylactic reactions. In patients with non-immunological contact urticaria it is often impossible to differentiate between contact urticarial and toxic reactions.

Several test procedures for contact urticaria are available:

- In vivo tests:
  - Open patch (application) test on healthy/affected skin
  - Occlusive patch and chamber test on healthy/affected skin
  - Prick, scratch, scratch-chamber test and intradermal test
- In vitro tests:
  - Detection of specific IgE – RAST etc.

The simplest in vivo diagnostic test for contact urticaria is the open patch (application) test.[7] In this test a small amount of the suspected substance is applied to skin of the back or the forearm.[2,3,8] Immunological contact urticaria reactions

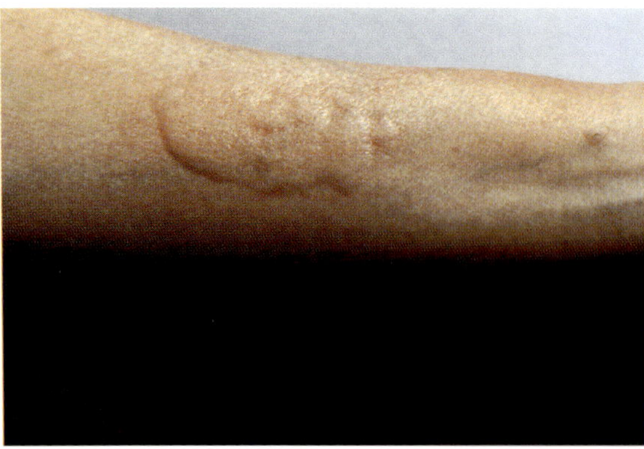

Figure 5.2: Contact urticaria to a chinolinolsulphate-containing cream.

can be expected within 15–20 min and non-immunological reactions within 45–60 min (with many exceptions from this rule!).

The occlusive patch and chamber tests are more sensitive than open application tests.[2] The patch chamber is removed after 15–20 min and a positive immunological reaction is to be expected immediately, but a non-immunological reaction often takes 10–40 min.[2,3]

Prick, scratch, scratch-chamber or intradermal tests may be used if the application or occlusive test results are negative.

The specific IgE level measured with RAST in serum correlates well with the results of the skin prick tests for most of the protein allergens.[9,10] However, RAST is unavailable for many potent contact allergens (Figure 5.2).

Contact urticaria from rubber

In 1979 Nutter[11] described the first case of contact urticaria to rubber gloves attributed to natural rubber (latex). Since this first report, many cases of IgE-mediated hypersensitivity reactions have been reported, including contact urticaria, rhinitis, conjunctivitis, asthma and anaphylaxis.[12–17]

Latex is the natural milky rubber sap obtained from the rubber tree, *Hevea brasiliensis*. Natural latex is the raw material for the manufacture of gloves, condoms, balloons and catheters, just to give a few examples. The use of articles containing natural rubber is widespread and this can explain the increasing frequency of allergic reactions to natural rubber latex. These reactions often affect healthcare and cleaning workers. The hazard for latex-allergic patients to react to a variety of fruits or plants is an additional problem based on true immunological cross reactions.[18,19]

Natural latex allergens are proteins present in the raw latex sap.[20] A number of these proteins are capable of binding IgE antibodies in sera from latex-allergic individuals. The so-called rubber elongation factor has recently been discussed as major allergen in this context. The natural latex allergens can be leached from gloves by normal skin moisture and are absorbed to the cornstarch powder. These cornstarch particles with absorbed latex allergen can become airborne and sensitize people by inhalation or produce symptoms such rhinitis and asthma in previously sensitized people.[21]

The most frequent symptoms are itching and burning with or without localized contact urticaria. Anaphylaxis is usually associated with parenteral or mucosal exposure. Reactions have occurred after contact with rubber bladder catheters or condoms, and dental procedures. Risk factors for sensitization to latex and diagnostic testing procedures are reviewed in detail later on in this book.

Protein contact dermatitis

In 1975, Hjorth and Roed-Petersen[7] reported a particular form of contact dermatitis under the name of "protein contact dermatitis" in 33 kitchen workers. In most cases these patients had eczema of the hands, with acute exacerbation when the skin was exposed to certain food proteins. Protein contact dermatitis is a chronic, recurrent dermatitis caused by contact with protein material.[22] Sometimes an urticarial or vesicular eruption is noted a few minutes after contact with the causative substance, and the reaction may be accompanied by pruritus, burning, stinging or pain.[23–29]

Most sources of protein contact dermatitis are occupational, such as food saps (fruit, vegetable, meat, flour), animal protein (bovine amniotic fluid), natural rubber latex or human protein fluids (Table 5.3). Consequently, food handlers, cooks, catering and kitchen workers, bakers and confectioners, veterinarians, and healthcare workers are the most likely to be affected.

Extracutaneous reactions such as abdominal cramps, diarrhoea, angioedema and pruritus or tingling of the oral mucosa may sometimes occur when the allergen is ingested.[25,28,30,31] When the allergen is volatile, allergic rhinoconjunctivitis and even bronchial asthma may accompany the skin reaction.[32–36] The protein contact dermatitis is often but not necessarily related to a personal or familial history of atopy. Usually, the lesions are confined to the hands and the forearms, because occupational allergens are by far the most important causes of protein contact dermatitis. However, depending upon the allergen, other sites may be affected.[25,26]

Protein contact dermatitis was thought to be a combination of type I and IV allergic reactions: type I because of the protein nature of the allergen, and type IV because of the eczematous nature of the lesion. A scratch-chamber test with the suspected material is commonly used to reveal the causative protein. Proteins, which are large molecules, cannot penetrate the skin unless it has be damaged. The scratch is required to enhance the absorption of high molecular weight material into the skin. This might be a reason why open tests on normal skin remain negative, whereas prick or scratch tests, in which the skin is damaged, produce an urticarial reaction a few minutes after application of the protein. Typically, there is an immediate-type wheal-and-flare reaction after 20–40 min, followed by a delayed-type skin reaction after 1–3 days, the real protein contact dermatitis. The latter is, however, often missing. Specific IgE may sometimes be detected in the serum and thereby adds to the diagnosis.

It may be that only a type I allergy to the suspected protein was involved in some of the cases described in the literature. The eczema could well have an irritant origin, or could be the result of a delayed allergic reaction. That delayed skin tests are often negative does not necessarily mean a delayed allergic reaction is not involved, as these results might be falsely negative.[37]

Table 5.3 Selected substances reported to cause protein contact dermatitis

Fruits, vegetables, spices, plants	*Animal proteins*
Almond	Amniotic fluid
Banana	Blood: pig, cow
Bean	Mesenteric fat: pig
Caraway	Liver: calf, chicken
Carrot	Meat: cow, pig, chicken, horse, lamb
Castor bean	Skin: chicken, turkey
Flower	Saliva: cow
Celery	Fish: cod, cuttlefish, herring, shrimps, lobster, mackerel
Chicory	Cheese: Cheddar, Emmental
Chrysanthemum	Egg yolk
Cress	Milk: cow
Cucumber	
Curry	*Grains*
Dill	Rye flour
Eggplant	Wheat flour
Endive	Barley flour
Fig	
Hazelnut	*Enzymes*
Horseradish	α-amylase
Kiwi fruit	
Lemon	
Lettuce	
Paprika	
Parsley	
Parsnip	
Peanuts	
Pineapple	
Potato	
Tomato	

Standardization of scratch-chamber tests is still in very early days. There is almost no commercially available test allergen; most allergists use prick or intradermal test solution or even native material if appropriate. When using native material, serial dilution and inclusion of a negative control such as the diluent are recommended. Irritant and weak reactions can be seen frequently, especially for flour, meat or high-ammonium latex milk. This is easy to understand because much live material contains enzymes or is subject to degradation under occlusive conditions on microbially contaminated skin.

We will learn more about this interesting type of contact dermatitis when we have reliable, reproducible, non-irritant test methods. Studies are needed to find out what test concentration has the highest sensitivity and reproducibility. So far, there remain many false-positive and false-negative results in our test protocols.

References

1. Kligmann AM, The spectrum of contact urticaria. Wheals, erythema, and pruritus. *Dermatol Clin* 1990; **8**:57–60.
2. Von Krogh, Maibach HI, The contact urticaria syndrome. *Semin Dermatol* 1982; **1**:59–66.
3. Lahti A, Non immunologic contact urticaria. *Acta Derm Venereol (Stockh)* 1980; **60**:(suppl 91).
4. Lahti A, Krogh G, Maibach HI, Contact urticaria syndrome. In: Stone J, ed. *Dermatologic Immunology and Allergy*. St Louis: Mosby; **28**:379–390.
5. Monroe EW, Urticaria. *Int J Dermatol* 1981; **20**:32–39.
6. Maibach HI, Johnson HL, Contact urticaria syndrome. Contact urticaria to diethyltoluamide (immediate type hypersensitivity). *Arch Dermatol* 1975; **111**:726–730.
7. Hjorth N, Roed-Petersen J. Occupational protein contact dermatitis in food handlers. *Contact Dermatitis* 1976; **2**:28–42.
8. Emmons WW, Marks JG Jr, Immediate and delayed reactions to cosmetic ingredients. *Contact Dermatitis* 1985; **13**:258–265.
9. Aas, K, Backman A, Belin L, Weeke B, Standardization of allergen extracts with appropriate methods. The combined use of skin prick testing and radio-allergosorbent test. *Allergy* 1978; **33**:130–137.
10. De Filippi I, Yman L, Schröder H, Clinical accuracy of updated version of the Phadrebas RAST® test. *Ann Allergy* 1981; **46**:249–255.
11. Nutter AE, Contact urticaria due to rubber. *Br J Dermatol* 1979; **101**:597–604.
12. Belsito DW, Contact urticaria caused by rubber. Analysis of seven cases. *Dermatol Clin* 1990; **8**:61–66.
13. Pecquet C, Leynadier F, Dry J, Contact urticaria and anaphylaxis to natural latex. *J Am Acad Dermatol* 1990; **22**:631–633.
14. Slater JE, Rubber anaphylaxis. *N Engl J Med* 1989; **320**:1126–1130.
15. Spaner D, Dolovich J, Tarlo S et al., Hypersensitivity to natural latex. *J Allergy Clin Immunol* 1989; **83**:1135–1137.
16. Tarlo SM, Wong L, Roos J et al., Occupational asthma caused by latex in a surgical glove manufacturing plant. *J Allergy Clin Immunol* 1990; **85**:626–631.

17. Taylor J, Evey P, Helm T et al., Contact urticaria and anaphylaxis from latex. *Contact Dermatitis* 1990; **23**:277–279.

18. Ahlroth M, Alenius H, Turjanmaa K et al., Cross-reacting allergens in natural rubber latex and avocado. *J Allergy Clin Immunol* 1995; **96**:167–172.

19. Carey AB, Cornish K, Schrank P et al., Cross-reactivity of alternate plant sources of latex in subjects with systemic IgE-mediated sensitivity to *Hevea brasiliensis* latex. *Ann Allergy Asthma Immunol* 1995; **74**:317–322.

20. Slater JE, Allergic reactions to natural rubber. *Ann Allergy* 1992; **68**:203–209.

21. Bubak ME, Reed CE, Fransway AF et al., Allergic reactions to latex among health-care workers. *Mayo Clin Proc* 1992; **67**:1075–1081.

22. Janssens V, Morren M, Dooms-Goossens A, Degreef H, Protein contact dermatitis: myth or reality? *Br J Dermatol* 1995; **132**:1–6.

23. Veien NK, Hattel T, Justesen O, Norholm A, Causes of eczema in the food industry. *Derm Beruf Umwelt* 1983; **31**:84–86.

24. Ninimäki A, Scratch-chamber tests in food handler dermatitis. *Contact Dermatitis* 1987; **16**:11–20.

25. Krook G. Occupational dermatitis from *Lactuca sativa* (lettuce) and *Cichorium* (endive). Simultaneous occurence of immediete and delayed allergy as a cause of contact dermatitis. *Contact Dermatitis* 1977; **3**:27–36.

26. Schirmer RH, Kalveram KJ, Kalveram CM et al., Chronisch lichenoide Dermatitis bei Sensibilisierung gegen Alphe-Amylase bei einem Bäcker. *Z Hautkr* 1987; **62**:792–797.

27. Rostenberg A, Contact urticaria from food. *Arch Dermatol* 1970; **101**:491–493.

28. Larkö O, Lindstedt G, Lundberg PA, Mobacken H, Biochemical and clinical studies in a case of contact urticaria to potato. *Contact Dermatitis* 1983; **9**:108–114.

29. Fisher AA, Stengel F, Allergic occupational hand dermatitis due to calf's liver. An urticarial "immediate" type hypersensitivity. *Cutis* 1977; **19**:561–565.

30. Fisher AA, Contact urticaria from handling meats and fowl. *Cutis* 1977; **19**:561–565.

31. Toby Mathias CG, Contact urticaria from peanut butter. *Contact Dermatitis* 1983; **9**:66–68.

32. Kanerva L, Estlander T, Jolanki R, Long-lasting contact urticaria. Type I and type IV allergy from castor bean and a hypotesis of systemic IgE-mediated allergic dermatitis. *Dermatol Clin* 1990; **8**:181–188.

33. Kanerva L, Estlander T, Jolanki R, Long-lasting contact urticaria from castor bean. *J Am Acad Dermatol* 1990; **23**:351–355.

34. Tarvainen K, Salonen JP, Kanerva L et al., Allergy and toxicodermia from shiitake mushroom. *J Am Acad Dermatol* 1991; **24**:64–66.

35. Morren M, Janssens V, Dooms-Goossens A, Alpha-amylase, a flour additive as an important cause of protein contact dermatitis in bakers. *J Am Acad Dermatol* 1993; **29**: 723–728.

36. Thomsen RJ, Honsinger RW, Immediate hypersensitivity reaction to amphibian serum manifesting as hand eczema. *Arch Dermatol* 1987; **123**:1436–1437.

37. Friedmann PS, Graded continuity, or all ornone-studies of the human immune response. *Clin Exp Dermatol* 1991; **16**:79–84.

38. Malten KE, The occurence of hybrids between contact allergic eczema and atopic dermatitis (and vice versa) and their significance. *Dermatologica* 1968; **136**:404–406.

39. Maibach H, Immediate hypersensitivity in hand dermatitis. *Arch Dermatol* 1976; **112**:1289–1291.

6. Systemic Contact Dermatitis

Matthias Gebhardt

Contact dermatitis is of course a reaction of eczematous morphology. However, in addition to dermatitis, non-eczematous reactions based on a type IV immune reaction can also occur and in these it is also wise to consider patch tests as a diagnostic tool. A wide variety of these cutaneous eruptions may be elicited by systemic uptake of an agent, usually a drug or food (Table 6.1), and are termed systemic contact dermatitis (SCD). It is not known whether the eruption is really a type IV allergy to the causative agent; other immunological mechanisms may also contribute. This may explain why fever, headaches and malaise are not uncommon upon re-exposure to the triggering agent.

Table 6.1 Substances reported in systemic contact dermatitis (SCD)

Substance	••	*Substance*	••
Food		Phenacone	CD
Spices, flavours, balsam of Peru	CD	Gold	CD
Sorbic acid	CD	Piroxicam	PCD
Garlic	CD	*Oral antidiabetics*	
Cashew nut oleoresins	CD	Sulphonyl urea derivatives	CD
		Complementary medicine	
Drugs		Chinese medicines	CD
Corticosteroids	CD	Tea tree oil	CD
Antibiotics		*Other*	
Gentamicin, neomycin	CD	Chloroquine	CD
Ampicillin	CD	Isoniazid	CD
Erythromycin	CD	Dimethyl sulphoxide	CD
Tricyclic antidepressants	PCD	Valium	CD
Antineoplastic agents		Quinine, quinidine	CD
Mitomycin C	CD	Disulfiram (Antabuse)	CD
5-Fluorouracil	CD		
Anti-allergic drugs		*Metals*	
Pseudoephidrine	CD	Mercury, dental amalgam	CD
Ethylendiamine	CD	Nickel	CD
Hydroxyzine	CD	Copper (intrauterine devices)	CD
Anaesthetics		Gold (as medication)	CD
Suxamethonium	CD		
Local anaesthetics	CD	*Miscellaneous*	
Doxepin cream	CD	Thiurams from hemodialysis unit	CD
Analgetics, antirheumatics		Rosin	CD
Hydromorphone	CD	Tea tree oil	CD

CD, contact dermatitis;
PCD, photocontact dermatitis

Table 6.2 Clinical appearance of systemic contact dermatitis (SCD)
Flare of previously positive patch test sites
Baboon syndrome
Involvement of the major folds
Vesicular hand eczema
Systemic symptoms: fever, malaise, headaches

Usually, the SCD spread symmetrically and is most pronounced in the major axillae and interdigital spaces and periorificially. Interestingly, previous lesions such as patch test fields or once eczematous areas readily flare up during the elicitation phase of SCD. Morphologically, the spreading dermatitis may be erythematous, like erythema multiforme, pustular, vesicular, pruritic, haemorrhagic or, not least, eczematous (Table 6.2).

Baboon syndrome is a special and probably the most typical form of SCD elicited by oral ingestion, injection or inhalation of the causative agent.[1] It is eruption arising in perianogenital skin and involves the inner thighs, giving the appearance of baboon in the same area. Patients with baboon syndrome may be suspected of having a textile dermatitis to underpants, which cover the area most severely affected. Several drugs, metals (nickel, mercury) and foods have been suspected for eliciting this type of SCD.

Foods

Many single case reports give evidence that foods can elicit contact dermatitis by systemic uptake. This is particularly true for foods that crossreact with common contact allergens. For example, some spices are related to ingredients of essential oils. **Cinnamon** is one of these. Commonly used to flavour baking goods, toothpaste, beverages such as cola and other soft drinks, cinnamon resembles a group of allergens that includes cinnamon oil, cinnamic aldehyde and cinnamic alcohol, which are responsible for the high incidence of contact allergy to balsam of Peru or fragrance mix.[2] Oral provocation with cinnamon is easily carried out to prove the relevance. Other spices of relevance include nutmeg, cardamom, curry, coriander, turmeric and laurel.[3] The crossreactivity between balsam of Peru and spices, flavourings, orange peel (in jam, soft drinks, liqueurs), vanilla, liquorice, etc., may induce a flare of dermatitis after eating or drinking the above-mentioned products.

Another possible type IV allergen in food is nickel from tin cans, pots and conserves, and nickel-containing food such as nuts, beans, peas and chocolate.

There has been some discussion of whether nickel-containing alloys may release significant amounts of nickel ions into foods or beverages and whether this nickel is capable of inducing skin eruptions similar to those attributed to nickel contact with the skin. In fact, oral nickel provocation with doses of up to 2.5mg has shown vesicular hand eczema and flare of formerly positive patch test sites. One criticism of this, however is that daily uptake of nickel via food is less than 2.5mg and that the consequence of nickel avoidance is hardly realized. It is interesting to find dermatitis flaring up upon nickel provocation, but the clinical appearance of the flare should be similar to that of the preceding eczema. Patch test positivity to nickel sulphate in less than 5% pet concentrations may be a good indicator of relevance for systemic nickel provocation as an eczema trigger.

Metals

Devices in subcutaneous tissue such as orthopaedic metals may elicit an eczematous eruption in the overlying skin which is, to some extent, also belonging to systemic contact dermatitis. **Mercury** exanthema in the typical distribution of SCD was observed by Nakayama et al.[4] in 15 patients. Using different sensitization methods, the flare was mainly elicited by efforts to collect the mercury particles from broken thermometers. Elevated temperatures were common accompanying signs in these patients. Patch testing revealed crossreactivity to several inorganic mercury compounds, and also to organic compounds to a lesser extent.

Not all mercury compounds are likely to cause flares following systemic uptake. An example of good tolerance despite a high rate of patch test positivity is thimerosal. This preservative is frequently used in vaccines and, as several studies have shown, many patients are sensitized by receiving vaccines preserved with thimerosal. However, upon revaccination, the vaccine is tolerated well in most cases, even though it contains thimerosal; hence giving vaccines that contain this allergen is recommended when no alternative is available (as in hepatitis B, FSME, influenza, etc.).

Allergy to **gold** salts is rather common. It is mostly a cross reaction in people who are allergic to nickel and has possible relevance in jewellery intolerance and dentistry. Gold sodium thiomalate is an antirheumatic agent given systemically by intramuscular injection; patients with contact allergy to gold had flares of the antecedent patch test site, rashes and/or fever following injection of this antirheumatic.[5]

Some comments about the relevance of **nickel** in food have been given earlier in this chapter and can be applied to nickel-containing alloys, such as those found in orthopaedic and dental materials. Further information is given in Chapter 14.

Drugs and medicaments

These are probably the most common elicitors of SCD. Further information about this topic is given in Chapter 8. There are plenty of single case reports, covering a wide range of pharmaceutical agents. It can be difficult to differentiate between real eczematous reactions and other types of maculopapular rashes; however, even the latter have been reproduced by patch testing possible causative drugs. One of the most interesting drugs is disulfiram (Antabuse), which is tetraethyl thiuram disulphide. This substance is also used in pesticides and in rubber. While sensitization to rubber chemicals is frequent, there is also a chance that patients who receive disulfiram will develop SCD.[6]

A crucial point in evaluating such cases is the mode of induction of SCD. The oral and intravenous routes are not the only modes of uptake of potential allergens, especially for pharmaceutical preparations. When taking a patient's history it is also important to ask about ophthalmic, rectal and vaginal preparations; over-the-counter drugs are frequently forgotten and the same is true for vaginal medications (indeed, systemic spread of a given drug has been attributed to absorption through the vaginal wall.)[7] Intravesical instillation of antitumour agents is a quite common mode of systemic induction of contact dermatitis – either palmoplantar appearance, genital spread or widespread eczematous lesions. Recently, I came across a case of an erythema multiforme like eruption of the upper trunk and arms secondary to use of a gentamicin-containing ophthalmic ointment; others have described erythema multiforme due to ophthalmic sulphonamides.

Crossreactivity is another aspect that has to be mentioned. Patients topically sensitized to neomycin should not be given kanamycin, streptomycin or gentamycin by any systemic route. There are many chemical relatives of the *para* group and when a patient is sensitized to any *para* substance topically (such as paraphenylenediamine, benzocaine, PABA sunscreens and diazo dyes), he or she is at (rare) risk of acquiring SCD by intake of sulphonylurea antidiabetics, sulphonamides, local anaesthetics of the PABA type (benzocaine in throat tablets, haemorrhoid and stomatitis preparations) or parabens used as preservatives in drugs.[2,8] Another well-known combination is that of rubber thiuram allergy and systemic provocation by disulfiram.

Table 6.3 gives a shortened list of drugs commonly associated with phototoxic effects. Sometimes, it is rather difficult to distinguish between **phototoxic** and **photoallergic reactions**. This is especially true for some NSAIDs. Only a detailed case history can determine the relevance of such a reaction. An allergic reaction to photoproducts of a given substance has been proposed as explanation in cases in which criteria of both phototoxicity and allergy are present.[10] Further information about phototoxic and photoallergic contact dermatitis is given in Chapter 18.

Table 6.3 Pharmaceutical agents with phototoxic properties[9]

Tricyclic antidepressants
Contraceptive steroids
Diphenhydramine
Chlorpromazine and other phenothiazines
Nifedipine
Chloramphenicol
Nitrofurantoin
Chlordiazepoxide
Olaquindox (veterinary medicine)
Methaqualone

A crucial aspect of systemically induced contact dermatitis is the question of whether systemic drugs may elicit reactions if the sensitization was acquired by topical treatment. Corticosteroids are a rare cause of both topical and SCD. In a study of patients sensitized by corticosteroid treatment of hand eczema, perianal eczema and vasculitis of the legs, systemic challenge caused not only flare of the preceding positive patch test sites but also flare of the previously affected sites. Interestingly, induction of endogenous cortisone following i.v. adrenocorticotrophic hormone application also elicited a delayed flare in one patient.[11]

References

1. Andersen KE, Hjorth N, Menne T, The baboon syndrome: systemically induced allergic contact dermatitis. *Contact Dermatitis* 1984; **10**:97–100.

2. Fisher AA, Systemic contact-type dermatitis due to drugs. *Dermatol Clinics* 1986; **4**:58–69.

3. Dooms-Goossens A, Dubelloy R, Degreef H, Contact and systemic contact-type dermatitis to spices. *Dermatol Clinics* 1990; **8**:89–93.

4. Nakayama H, Niki F, Shono M, Hada S, Mercury exanthem. *Contact Dermatitis* 1983; **9**:411–417.

5. Larssen A, Mölller H, Björkner B et al., Morphology of endogenous flare-up reactions in contact allergy to gold. *Acta Derm Venereol (Stockh)* 1997; **77**:474–479.

6. Menne T, Veien NK, Maibach HI, Systemic contact-type dermatitis due to drugs. *Semin Dermatol* 1989; **8**:144–148.

7. Goette DK, Odom RB, Vaginal medications as a cause for varied widespread dermatitides. *Cutis* 1980; **26**:406–409.

8. Carradori S, Peluso AM, Faccioli M, Systemic contact dermatitis due to parabens. *Contact Dermatitis* 1990; **22**:238–239.

9. Beijersbergen van Henegouwen GMJ, (Systemic) phototoxicity of drugs and other xenobiotics. *J Photochem Photobiol B* 1991; **10**:183–210.

10. Hölzle E, Neumann N, Hausen B et al., Photopatch testing: the 5-year experience of the German, Austrian and Swiss Photopatch Test Group. *J Am Acad Dermatol* 1991; **25**:59–68.

11. Lauerma AI, Reitamo S, Maibach HI, Systemic hydrocortisone/cortisone induces allergic skin reactions in presensitized subjects. *J Am Acad Dermatol* 1991; **24**:182–185.

7. Contact Allergy in Atopic Dermatitis

Matthias Gebhardt

Atopic dermatitis (AD) is a heterogeneous disease. The course and clinical picture change not only with age but also from patient to patient (Figures 7.1 to 7.3). Therefore, general conclusions are likely to deceive the dermatologist. Three different factors regarding contact dermatitis in AD should be stressed:

- Aeroallergen-induced contact dermatitis
- Allergic contact dermatitis (ACD) in AD
- Irritant contact dermatitis in AD

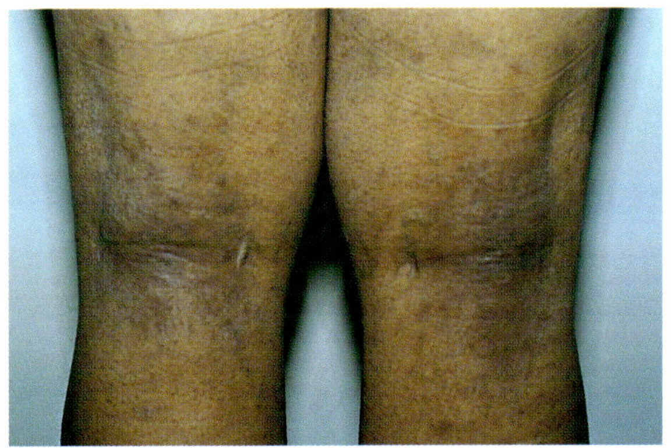

Figure 7.1: Typical flexural atopic eczema.

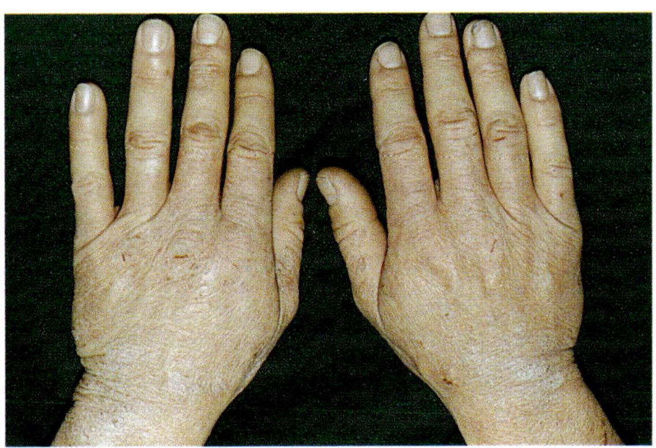

Figure 7.2: Irritant contact dermatitis of the hands due to soaps and detergents.

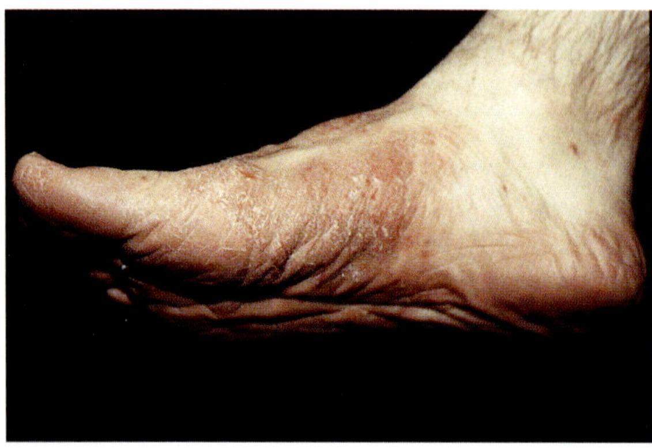

Figure 7.3: Atopic foot eczema.

Aeroallergen-induced contact dermatitis

House dust mites, pollens, moulds and animal dander have been found to aggravate the course of atopic eczema. These and other aeroallergens quite often cause contact urticarial responses in AD due to specific IgE sensitization. However, their role in eliciting eczematous reactions still remains doubtful. The various opinions have been put into three different categories, seeing aeroallergens:

- as a major cause
- as a triggering factor
- without relevance

Reasons for assuming that type I allergens have a role in AD are:

- high incidence of elevated serum IgE
- associated asthma, allergic rhinitis and urticaria
- multiple positive prick reactions to inhalant allergens
- elevated serum and urinary histamine (possibly from mast cell degranulation)

In order to prove a role for aeroallergens in eliciting eczematous reactions, the **aeroallergen patch test** was devised in the early 1980s.

Epidermal Langerhans cells are found to bear the IgE receptor, both of the high- and the low-affinity type.[1,2] IgE-bearing Langerhans cells are able to present aeroallergens that have been absorbed by the skin. It is hard to believe that large proteins such as house dust mite (HDM) allergens, pollens and animal dander can enter the skin. However, Maeda et al. showed that HDM allergens can indeed penetrate the epidermis and bind to Langerhans cells.[3] Bruijnzeel-

Koomen et al.[4] were able to demonstrate that only IgE-bearing Langerhans cells are capable of presenting those allergens. However, Bieber et al.[2] have demonstrated that IgE-bearing Langerhans cells are not specific for AD, they occur in psoriasis and T-cell lymphoma as well. T Cells from the blood stream leave the blood vessels and migrate into the tissue mediated by adhesion molecules, among them CD4+ T cells of the T helper (Th) 0 type. These or more specialized Th2 cells recognize the allergen and proliferate. They produce cytokines of the Th2 type with specific actions, such as interleukin (IL) 4, the IgE upregulating lymphokine, and IL-5, the eosinophil chemotactic, and growth factors. In this model, AD is considered to be something like an IgE-mediated allergic contact eczema.[5] Recently, Grewe et al.[6] have shown that acute eczematous reactions are characterized by a Th2 pattern, but later on Th1 cytokines like IFN-γ dominate in atopic skin. This observation is problematic in terms of the current model of AD as a Th2-type skin disease and beg the question "What is the critical point of the aeroallergen patch test?".

Most procedures used in the aeroallergen patch test are highly irritant to atopic skin, for example tape stripping, scratching or using very high protein concentrations under occlusive conditions for about 2 days. Aeroallergen patch tests need to be standardized; in their current form they are not in any way a "gold standard" of allergen identification in AD. Nevertheless early results have shown that aeroallergen patch tests are rather reliable. The tests can now be performed on normal uninvolved skin without artificial manipulation such as tape stripping or use of irritants and they have been standardized regarding the use of vehicle and dose–response relationships.[7] HDM patch tests in a large group of AD patients has shown a 21% positivity compared with 0.75% in controls. Interestingly, positive patch tests are not always accompanied by positive immediate-type reactions to mites.[8]

In my opinion, there are eczematous reactions to aeroallergens. However, whether these reactions are the product of a Th2-type contact dermatitis or the sequelae of urticarial reactions has yet to be shown. Urticarial responses to type I allergens occurring in eczematous regions that are already red and itchy are attributed to the eczema instead of contact urticaria. Increased scratching might be followed by eczematization. Four requirements for the proof of an allergen cause for AD have been published recently by Hanifin and Klas:[9]

- maintenance/worsening of the disease when the environment contains the suspected allergen
- clearing/improvement in an allergen-free environment
- morphologically and histologically similar lesions consistently reproduced by epicutaneous skin-test application of purified allergen
- disease extent and distribution reproduced by challenge with purified allergen

Considering these factors, we shall be able to improve our understanding of the role of type I allergy in AD.

There are several current studies regarding aeroallergen standardization for patch test purposes. HDMs are already available for patch test purposes; other aeroallergens will follow soon. More well-prepared epidemiological studies are now required to give us a more sophisticated picture of the true role of aeroallergens in "atopic contact dermatitis".

Allergic contact dermatitis in AD

Until recently we were taught in dermatology that ACD is less common in AD patients than in non-atopics. This observation was mainly based on experimental sensitization studies with dinitrochlorobenzene (DNCB) on AD skin, showing decreasing rates of sensitization to DNCB with increasing severity of the skin disease.[10] Meanwhile, many other studies have given contradictory results.

Motolese et al.[11] found higher sensitization rates in atopic children than in non-atopics. Although another large survey of almost 1000 patients by Cronin and McFadden[12] did not confirm a higher rate of contact allergies in atopics, there are indeed considerable numbers of contact allergic patients among AD patients. Fragrance and nickel allergics have been found in the same frequency in all groups, indicating that at least for these two allergens atopics are not less likely to become sensitized. This observation was confirmed by another study by the same group on hairdressers with hand dermatitis.[13] Patients with atopic manifestations in either skin or mucous membranes had the same contact allergy frequency and the same allergen rank as non-atopics.

In a large Finnish study[14] atopic individuals were patch tested. Nickel, fragrance mix, balsam of Peru and neomycin were the commonest allergens in all groups, not only in AD but also in atopic airway diseases! As expected, contact allergy to topical medicaments was common among AD patients. Patients with severe and long-lasting dermatitis were most frequently sensitized. The authors tried to minimize irritant effects by additionally testing 50% dilutions of the test substances, which did not solve the problem. A recent Egyptian study found neomycin to be more frequent among hand dermatitis patients with elevated IgE than in those without.[15]

Reviewing all the data enables us to summarize the current state of knowledge. There is a less frequent rate of contact sensitization in AD patients than might be expected in view of their disturbed epidermal protection against environmental chemicals, their use of multiple topical substances and their skin inflammation. Nevertheless, the statement that AD patients are unable to generate ACD reactions because of their specific T-cell defect is all but true. Nickel, the fragrance group and neomycin seem to be leading allergens among these patients.

However, there are many problems in interpreting the data:

- Some cases of ACD might be misinterpreted as AD because of the similar clinical pattern of disease. For example, reactions to plant allergens such as Compositae, or airborne contact sensitization to resin, cement dust or formaldehyde, are very likely to mimic AD, and ACD to textiles can give the same clinical picture such as AD (flexural eczema).
- Patch tests on atopic skin may give false-positive reactions because of increased skin irritability. This is especially true for metals, which are likely to cause follicular pustular reactions. The confirmation of relevance is crucial in these cases, especially important in medicolegal cases of occupational dermatology where we have to decide between pre-existing conditions (atopy) and occupation-related triggers (allergens). The confirmation or rejection of a diagnosis of contact sensitization has a dramatic influence on the social status of the affected person.
- True patch test reactions may be suppressed by immunosuppressive therapeutic measures, both topical and systemic. This will become more and more important in the future when potent immunosuppressives will be available for AD (for example FK 506 and cyclosporin A).

For practical reasons, one should consider patch tests in AD whenever a skin disease is getting worse despite sufficient treatment. A good example is provided by topical medications used to treat AD: corticosteroids, for example, are crucial allergens to discover. When they are used to treat eczema, if the condition worsens because of contact allergy to the treatment, patients are likely to apply more ointment and the skin disorder deteriorates even more. Tixocortol pivalate and hydrocortisone-17-butyrate have been proposed as markers of corticosteroid allergy, but the patient's own steroid creams should always be included in tests. Late patch test readings are required not to miss delayed patch test reactions.[16] Table 7.1 lists some of the allergens that are of special importance in AD.

Irritant contact dermatitis

Very similar to the ACD problem are irritants as triggering factors of AD. There are three different ways in which irritation may be important:

- Atopic skin is more readily subject to irritation than healthy skin
- Irritants are a possible cause of false-positive patch test reactions, which in turn may be misleading
- Preventive (e.g. gloves) and therapeutic (e.g. lotions, creams) measures may also be irritating to atopic skin

Table 7.1 Allergens with relevance for atopic dermatitis

Nickel	Involved in many cases of dyshidrotic hand eczema; also systemic nickel ingestion
Fragrances	Fragrance mix is the most frequent allergen in latest data. Weak positive fragrance mix reactions are quite often of irritant nature, which may be a particular problem in AD patients. Sensitization rates to fragrances are similar in AD patients, mucosal atopy patients and controls; despite a lower rate for all contact allergens in the first group[13]
Topical medications	Neomycin, bufexamac, corticosteroids
Compositae	Airborne contact dermatitis to Compositae is a major differential diagnosis in AD
Natural rubber latex	Protein contact dermatitis is probably the fastest increasing problem in allergy
Aeroallergens	Causative role in AD is shown in many studies on aeroallergen patch test positivity, avoidance studies and supported by high levels of aeroallergen-specific IgE

Irritants in occupations, hobbies, skin treatment, cosmetics and in the house complicate AD cases. An increased cutaneous reactivity in AD may result from impaired epidermal barriers, increased expression of cellular adhesion molecules and lymphokines, and chronic exposure to skin care products and medications. A major problem arising from cutaneous irritability in AD is the problem of impaired occupational health. Many occupations are less appropriate for AD patients, especially occupations with a higher share of irritants such as wet work, dust, chemical or biological hazards. Therefore, professions such as those given in Table 7.2 are not favourable for skin atopics.

Summary

Taken together, most AD cases are influenced by environmental factors, not infrequently irritants. ACD is a possible co-factor, complication and differential diagnosis of AD. Contact dermatitis in AD patients is a particular problem in occupational dermatology. Therefore, some professions are not recommendable for individuals with active atopic skin disease. Recalcitrant courses of AD might be explained by development of ACD reactions to topical drugs used in dermatology. Some IgE-mediated allergens are of special interest in AD management: latex and, probably, mites, animal dander, moulds and pollens. These may be real "IgE-mediated contact allergens".

Table 7.2 Professions less suitable for AD patients

Hairdresser
Health care workers, medical nurses, medical doctor, dentist, veterinary personnel
Cleaner
Laboratory worker (chemistry, medicine)
Metalworker
Construction worker
Painter
Ceramic worker
Carpenter
Cook, caterer, food processor or handler
Florists, gardener
Farmer

References

1. Bruijnzeel-Koomen C, van der Donk EM, Bruynzeel PL et al., Associated expression of CD1 antigen and Fc receptor for IgE on epidermal Langerhans cells from patients with atopic dermatitis. *Clin Exp Immunol* 1988; **74**:137–142.

2. Bieber T, Dannenberg B, Prinz JC et al., Occurrence of IgE-bearing epidermal Langerhans cells in atopic eczema: a study of the time course of the lesions and with regard to the IgE serum level. *J Invest Dermatol* 1989; **92**:215–219.

3. Maeda K, Yamamoto K, Tanaka Y et al., House dust mite (HDM) antigen in naturally occurring lesions of atopic dermatitis (AD): the relationship between HDM antigen in the skin and HDM antigen-specific IgE antibody. *J Dermatol Sci* 1992; **3**:73–77.

4. Bruijnzeel-Koomen CA, Mudde GC, Bruijnzeel PL, The presence of IgE molecules on epidermal Langerhans cells in atopic dermatitis and their significance for its pathogenesis. *Allerg Immunol Paris* 1989; **21**:219–223.

5. van Reijsen FC, Bruijnzeel-Koomen CAFM, Kalthoff F et al., Skin derived T cell clones of the Th2 phenotype in patients with atopic dermatitis. *J Allergy Clin Immunol* 1992; **90**:184–193.

6. Grewe M, Walther S, Gyufko K et al., Analysis of the cytokine pattern expressed in situ in inhalant allergen patch test reactions of atopic dermatitis patients. *J Invest Dermatol* 1995; **105**:407–410.

7. Ring J, Darsow U, Gfesser M, Vieluf D, The atopy patch test in evaluating the role of aeroallergens in atopic eczema. *Int Arch Allergy Immunol* 1997; **113**:379–383.

8. Castelain M, Birnbaum J, Castelain PY et al., Patch test reactions to mite antigens. A GERDA multicentre study. *Contact Dermatitis* 1993; **29**:246–250.

9. Hanifin JM, Klas P, The spectrum of cutaneous patch-test reactions in patients with atopic dermatitis. *Clin Rev Allergy Immunol* 1996; **14**:225–240.

10. Uehara M, Sawai T, A longitudinal study of contact sensitivity in patients with atopic dermatitis. *Arch Dermatol* 1989; **125**:366–368.

11. Motolese A, Manzini BM, Donini M, Patch testing in infants. *Am J Contact Dermatitis* 1995; **6**:153.

12. Cronin E, McFadden JP, Patients with atopic eczema do become sensitized to contact allergens. *Contact Dermatitis* 1993; **28**:225–228.

13. Sutthipisal N, McFadden JP, Cronin E, Sensitization in atopic and non-atopic hairdressers with hand eczema. *Contact Dermatitis* 1993; **29**:206–209.

14. Lammintausta K, Kalimo K, Fagerlund VL, Patch test reactions in atopic patients. *Contact Dermatitis* 1992; **26**:234–240.

15. el-Samahy MH, el-Kerdani T, Value of patch testing in atopic dermatitis. *Am J Contact Dermatitis* 1997; **8**:154–157.

16. Dooms-Goosens AE, Degreef HJ, Marien KJC, Coopman SA, Contact allergy to corticosteroids: a frequently missed diagnosis? *J Am Acad Dermatol* 1989; **21**:538–543.

8. Allergic Drug Reactions

Matthias Gebhardt

Allergic reactions on the skin are among the most frequent side-effects of drug therapy. Because of an individual's allergic sensitization, the allergic rash will relapse whenever the causative drug is given again later in life. Therefore, evaluation of the causes may be necessary to improve the spectrum of drugs available for the individual and to prevent further harmful effects.

Certain drugs cause defined cutaneous syndromes. These include iodides and bromides, hydantoins, corticosteroids, antimalarial agents, gold, cancer chemotherapeutic agents, tetracyclines, thiazides and sulphonamides, non-steroidal anti-inflammatory agents, and coumarin.[1] However, almost every drug can induce any kind of allergic reaction. Among these reactions, eczematous drug rashes are rather uncommon; most skin eruptions appear non-eczematous. This chapter should be read together with Chapter 6 on systemic contact dermatitis, which is a closely related subject. In the present chapter, drug-induced aggravation of pre-existing skin conditions such as acne, psoriasis and lichen planus are not discussed. Induction of skin disorders such as lupus erythematsus, scleroderma and others is also not within the scope of this book.

Serious drug reactions

Anyone who carries out patch tests or any other skin test should always keep in mind that serious adverse reactions can be induced by exposure to the test substance itself during the patch test.[2]

Lyell's syndrome (toxic epidermal necrolysis)

Lyell's syndrome (Figure 8.1) is the most harmful drug reaction, with potentially life-threatening skin and mucosal involvement. Large areas of the skin are necrotic and affected in the same way as in severe bullous burns. Differential diagnosis includes almost exclusively staphylococcal scalded skin syndrome (SSSS), which occurrs usually in infancy or childhood and is caused by toxic effects of epidermolysin, a toxin produced by *Staphylococcus aureus* type II 71. An immediate biopsy may differentiate between the two diseases, with necrosis of the entire epidermis in Lyell's syndrome but cleavage within the upper epidermis in SSSS. For a comprehensive review on Lyell's syndrome, see the excellent paper by Rojeau et al.[3]

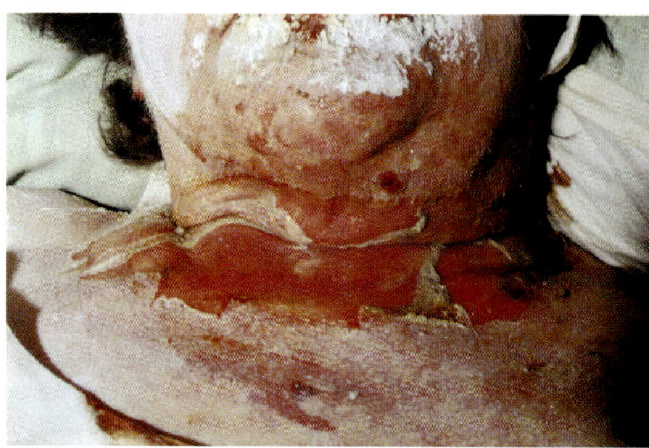

Figure 8.1: Lyell's syndrome.

The following drugs have been found more often to be associated with Lyell's syndrome:

- Non-steroidal anti-inflammatory drugs (NSAIDs)
- Antibiotics (sulphonamides)
- Anticonvulsants
- Allopurinol

There are in fact other non-pharmaceutical causes of toxic epidermal necrolysis, such as viral infections and immunizations, but sometimes those factors contribute to a drug aetiology masked by the manifestations of a viral infection.[4]

Erythema multiforme major

This is rather similar to Lyell's syndrome and some authors treat both diseases as the same entity. However, the intensity of the inflammatory infiltrate enables the pathologist to differentiate between the two disorders; there is a more intense inflammatory cellular infiltrate in erythema multiforme major.[5] There is a minor form of erythema multiforme which should not regarded as serious; initially it resembles urticaria in its clinical features, with subsequent development of a "target-like" picture. The acute development of target-like maculae on the skin along with extensive involvement of the mucosa is, however, characteristic of erythema multiforme major. Two different causes have to be taken into consideration: (post)herpes virus infection and drug intolerance. While treatment of the former with virustatics usually gives good results, the latter requires life-long avoidance of the possible causative drugs. In drug-induced erythema multiforme, however, patch tests may be indicated because of the strong T-cell infiltrate.[6] In some cases, it may be justifiable to perform patch tests with the suspected drugs. In my department, we have only done so with strict attention to the points given in Table 8.1.

Exfoliate dermatitis erythroderma[7]

This is another mostly drug-induced skin condition similar to toxic epidermal necrolysis (TEN) and Stevens–Johnson syndrome (SJS). It has to be differentiated from other causes of erythroderma such as T-cell lymphoma, psoriasis, toxic shock syndrome, atopic and seborrhoic dermatitis, etc. Differential diagnosis is based on the history and sudden onset of the drug-induced condition. Angiotensin-converting enzyme (ACE) inhibitors, anticonvulsants, ketoconazole and antibiotics have been described as inductors, similar to TEN and SJS.

Classification of severe drug reactions

Recently, Rojeau[6] published a paper suggesting a new classification for TEN, SJS and erythema multiforme based on their morphological distribution. In this scheme, the diagnosis of erythema multiforme, with or without mucosal involvement, requires target-like lesions and predominantly acral involvement, whereas SJS and TEN are considered to be similar disorders arising in central parts of the body, forming bullae on discrete macules and showing epidermal necrosis. Approximately 50% of erythema multiforme cases have herpes virus pathogenesis whereas SJS and TENS are almost always drug related.[6]

Anticonvulsant hypersensitivity syndrome

Anticonvulsants such as phenytoin, carbamazepine and phenobarbitone have been linked recently to a rare syndrome that is more than just a skin disease and has some clinical similarities with the above-mentioned skin syndromes. The triad of fever, skin rash and lymphadenopathy starting a few weeks after initiation of therapy is characteristic and should always make the clinician suspicious.[8]

Table 8.1 Criteria that must be fulfilled before patch testing in the evaluation of serious drug rashes
More than one previously taken drug must be under suspicion
The drug is hard to avoid or replace
The skin condition is not life threatening
The patient must be observed in a clinical setting for 5 days after application of the patch test (reactions may occur very late!)
The patient must give his/her thoroughly informed consent to the re-exposure

A variety of other target organs may be involved, including the liver, kidneys and lungs. In contrast to other types of drug intolerance, patch tests and lymphocyte stimulation assays are frequently positive in carbamazepine-induced hypersensitivity syndrome.[9] A 1% pet preparation of carbamazepine has been found useful for patch test purposes.[10]

Non-serious drug reactions

Acute generalized exanthematous pustulosis (AGEP)

This is a particular form of pustular drug eruption also referred to as pustular toxicoderm. Macrolide and β-lactam antibiotics are the main causes but diltiazem and nystatin[11] have also been reported. It has to be differentiated from pustular psoriasis and other pustular skin disorders. Leucocytosis and fever are common clinical signs in AGEP. Patch testing has been tried in order to establish the causative drug and has revealed a positive reaction in some cases. AGEP may be put on the borderline between a serious and a non-serious drug eruption, and hence strict caution is required when doing patch test re-exposure in these patients.

Drug rashes of urticarial, macular or papular appearance

These are commonly but not always accompanied by viral infection, mostly of the respiratory tract. The pathogenesis may be based on immunological and non-immunological mechanisms. HIV infection is a common co-factor for trimethoprim–sulphamethoxazole drug rashes. This sulphonamide is important for the prevention of opportunistic infections. Therefore, it is very helpful that successful desensitization protocols have been developed.[12,13] The nature of the drug rashes in HIV infection – allergic or toxic – is still doubtful.

A morbilliform exanthema after treatment of tonsillitis/pharyngitis with ampicillin or amoxicillin is almost diagnostic for Epstein–Barr virus infection and has been reported to occur in approximately 90% of all cases with this combination. It is characteristic but misleading that the interval between treatment initiation and appearance of the first signs of the rash may be as long as 14 days. Thus treatment has sometimes already been cancelled before the allergic reaction begins. In my experience, morbilliform drug-induced rashes are not a good indication for patch testing because it almost always fails to yield positive reactions. In urticarial rashes patch or open patch testing may be recommended because the test is the least dangerous challenge method. Readings should be performed after 20 min, because of the immediate type of the reaction. Later readings may be successful after 6h and thereafter, as is usual in patch tests. Subsequently, scratch tests, intradermal tests and even some in vitro procedures may be indicated; this is, however, beyond the scope of this book.

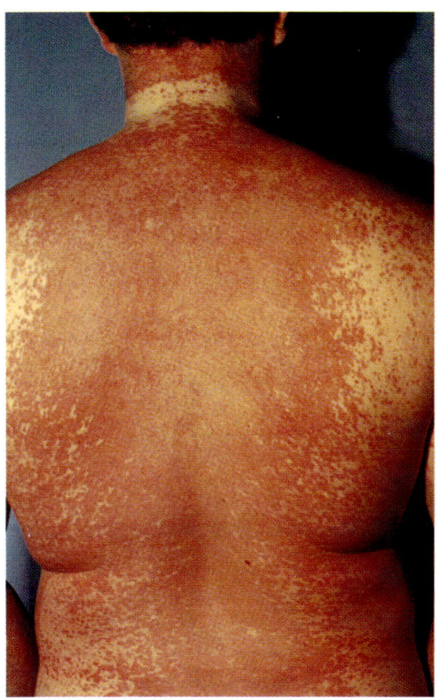

Figure 8.2: Macular exanthema after amoxicillin treatment.

Among common antibiotics, tetracycline has been found to be a more frequent elicitor (per number of prescriptions) of allergic skin reactions than minocycline or doxycycline (Figure 8.2).[14]

Eczematous plaques

Subcutaneous heparin injection is often associated with the appearance of eczematous infiltrated plaques. Histological examination shows dermatitis, dermal oedema and perivascular lymphocytic infiltration depending on the depth of the injection.[15] There is no general rule about the crossreactivity of one heparin to another. Decisions should be based on subcutaneous provocation of a panel of heparins, including high and low molecular weight heparins. It is my experience, in accordance with others, that patch tests and most intracutaneous tests fail to give positive reactions. Subcutaneous provocation followed by readings of the injection sites after 20 min and 1, 2 and 3 days is the diagnostic method of choice.

Mycosis fungoides-like plaques

Anticonvulsants such as phenytoin and carbamazepine have been associated with a peculiar mycosis fungoides-like eruption. Complete clearance occurs within a couple of weeks of discontinuation of the drug.[16]

Lichenoid reactions

There are two different ways in which lichenoid reactions can be elicited by systemic drugs. First, pre-existing lichen ruber can be aggravated by some drugs. Second, other agents may induce lichenoid changes. Among those commonly associated with lichenoid eruptions are β-blocking agents. When quinacrine hydrochloride was used for prevention of malaria a large number of lichenoid eruptions used to occur.[17]

Fixed drug eruption

Although never dangerous, this kind of intolerance reaction to a drug may be annoying because of burning or itching sensations. It resembles one or several sharply demarcated red to violet spots surrounded by normal skin. The macula may be infiltrated, flat or even evolve into a blister. The glans penis, perianal skin and oral mucosa are frequently involved but any region of the skin may be affected. After discontinuation of the drug the skin eruption persists for a while as pigmented maculae before disappearing. When a patient presents with a fixed drug eruption it may be helpful to take a photograph because later testing may be successful only within the borders of the previously affected skin area. A carefully taken history is most likely to reveal the causative agent, and allergy testing is avoidable in a high percentage of cases. If testing is necessary, I recommend starting with a patch test on the back as usual, followed by a scratch test on the arms and a scratch test within the earlier focus, step by step, until the test reaction is positive. The focal scratch test should optimally be read after 20 min and 6 and 24 h, to avoid missing a reaction. Drugs likely to be associated with fixed drug eruptions are NSAIDs, sedatives, laxatives and some antibiotics, e.g. sulphonamides (Figure 8.3).

Autoimmune progesterone dermatitis

This is an eczematous condition in females and also includes pruritus, urticaria and bullous erythema multiforme-like features. Typically it relapses, with close correlation to the second half of the menstrual cycle. A similar condition has been described for oestrogens.[18]

Primary induction by oral administration of synthetic steroids has been proposed[19] but refused by others. Currently, most authors recommend intradermal testing of progesterone; however, patch tests with 17-α-OH-progesterone 2% pet have failed to elicit a positive reaction.[20] I would first perform a patch test using progesterone 5% pet, followed by intradermal tests when the patch test is negative.

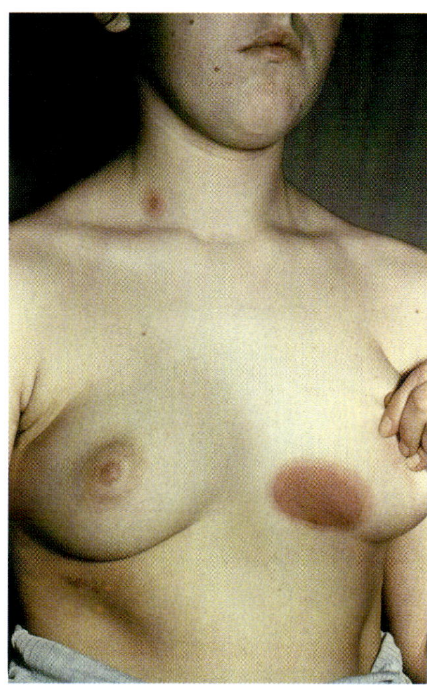

Figure 8.3: Fixed drug eruption.

Transdermal drug delivery systems (TDDS)

More and more agents are available in TDDS. It is important to differentiate irritant effects (e.g. tape adhesive irritation) and pharmacological effects (e.g. erythema from nitroglycerin), from real allergic reactions.[21] Only the latter require allergy management including diagnostics. When testing patients with previous eczematous reactions to TDDS, it is recommended that the producer of the TDDS is asked for a "dummy" sample free of the active agent to exclude irritant or allergic effects of the adhesive. In addition to local effects, TDDS is theoretically able to elicit a systemic drug rash by releasing considerable doses of the substance.

Crossreactivity and topical versus systemically induced contact dermatitis

An interesting example of crossreactivity has been repeatedly documented between thimerosal, namely the thiosalicylic acid part of the compound, and piroxicam. So, people with contact sensitization to thimerosal should be careful when taking piroxicam. Piroxicam, in this case, is a photoallergen. Another well-known problem is cross reaction between contact allergy to thiurams and systemic drug eruption to the drug disulfiram (Antabuse), given for alcoholism.

There is always much discussion as to whether to avoid systemic use of agents when there is contact allergy to these substances. Aminoglycoside antibiotics and chloramphenicol are good examples of this dilemma. It is not always proven that contact allergy to topical gentamycin, etc., leads to systemic elicitation of skin eruptions after oral or intravenous administration. However, case reports such as erythroderma in a neomycin contact allergic patient who developed erythroderma after i.v. gentamycin make it advisable to avoid all cross reactants by either a topical or systemic route.[22] Overall, one should avoid any re-exposure for medical or judicial reasons except for diagnostic purposes.

Patch tests for evaluation of drug rashes

As long as our understanding of drug rashes is not sufficiently comprehensive to produce well-established immunological indicators, the most reliable diagnostic tools remain in vivo re-exposure. Herein, patch testing a drug is a rather safe way of re-exposure. This is the main reason for using patch tests in the evaluation of skin rashes that occurred earlier. Of course, there are also severe, even fatal, reactions upon epicutaneous re-exposure to certain drugs, e.g. penicillin. However, as long as there is no proven standard in vitro test for the evaluation of allergic drug reactions, we have to rely on patch testing as the safest available test.

Despite some promising results reported as single cases or small studies, the patch test is not suitable for investigating every type of drug reaction. This is because of the various different mechanisms that may contribute to allergic and pseudoallergic drug reactions. T-cell involvement, as in patch testing, is a major part of our current concept of drug reaction but there is certainly more to it than that. The frequent appearance of drug rashes in all stages of HIV infection and in T-cell immunosuppressive lymphoma chemotherapy, affecting mainly CD4+ T cells, is just one argument against this well-accepted concept. However, for the management of some patients, patch test results may help to some extent.

Drug eruptions with a possible cellular basis include lichenoid reactions, SJS, toxic epidermal necrolysis, fixed drug eruption and lupus erythematosus-like conditions. In these, the patch test may be successful.[23] In my experience, patch tests are mostly disappointing in previous maculopapular rashes and of course, due to their lack of type IV nature, in urticarial rashes. Some specific drugs are more likely to cause a positive reaction, such as anticonvulsant drugs, some antibiotics, corticosteroids, ACE inhibitors and antirheumatics. In patients with allergic reactions to carbamazepine, 20% were patch test positive to carbamazepine in one study,[24] which is a rather high rate compared with other drugs. Other drugs are generally poor reactors on skin, such as neuroleptics, aspirin, narcotics and many others. For others, such as the heparins, the test substance should be applied subcutaneously and the test site skin read according to patch test criteria (i.e. after 1–3 days). However, there is no general rule due to the chemical nature of the medicaments whether to try or avoid patch tests with one or the other drug. Careful evaluation of further studies will at some time enable us to produce well-evaluated guidelines for the patch testing of systemic drugs, something which is unfortunately not possible at present.

The photo patch test should always be considered when the distribution of a drug eruption suggests a predominance of sun-exposed areas. The minimal erythema dose will be elevated in most of these cases, as long as the drug is systemically given, and will return to normal when avoided.

Oral, intra- or subcutaneous, or even intravenous challenge tests should be applied if a positive skin test reaction occurs and the tolerability of the non-reacting agents can be proved only by re-exposure. If one single drug is considered to be the cause, and in severe drug reactions, I would agree with most allergists that challenge tests are absolutely contraindicated.

Table 8.2 Reasons for negative patch test results with drug agents

Previous reaction not T-cell mediated
Lacking co-factor on re-exposure (virus, co-exposure to two different drugs, etc.)
Previous reaction to metabolite but not to original agent
Wrong test concentration
Wrong vehicle
Different way of antigen presentation

The most crucial problem in patch testing a drug is preparation of the test substances. So far, in terms of systemic drugs, there is almost nothing commercially available for patch tests. I have obtained useful results using a powdered and moisturized tablet or the powder from a capsule whenever the original purified agent was not easily available from pharmacies or by the company. Liquids can be taken as is if no particular recommendation is available for test concentrations. Some test concentrations are given in De Groot's tables.[25] It is recommended that at least 10 healthy controls are tested to exclude false-positive reactions, which is not easily done in daily practice. Table 8.2 lists a few examples of reasons for the lack of success of patch testing in the evaluation of drug rashes.

References

1. Wintroub BU, Stern R, Cutaneous drug reactions: pathogenesis and clinical classification. *J Am Acad Dermatol* 1985; **13**:167–179.

2. O'Donell BF, Tan CY, Erythema multiforme reaction to patch testing. *Contact Dermatitis* 1992; **27**:230–234.

3. Rojeau JC, Chosidow O, Saiag P, Guillaume JC, Toxic epidermal necrolysis (Lyell's syndrome). *J Am Acad Dermatol* 1990: **23**:1039–1058.

4. Avakian R, Flowers FP, Araujo OE, Ramos-Caro FA, Toxic epidermal necrolysis: a review. *J Am Acad Dermatol* 1991; **25**:69–79.

5. Paquet P, Pierard GE, Erythema multiforme and toxic epidermal necrolysis: a comparative study. *Am J Dermopathol* 1997; **19**:127–133.

6. Roujeau JC, Stevens–Johnson syndrome and toxic epidermal necrolysis are severity variants of the same disease which differs from erythema multiforme. *J Dermatol* 1997; **24:**726–729.

7. Breathnach SM, Management of drug eruptions: Part II. Diagnosis and treatment. *Aust J Dermatol* 1995; **36**:187–91.

8. Morkunas AR, Miller MB, Anticonvulsant hypersensitivity syndrome. *Crit Care Clin* 1997; **13**:727–739.

9. De Vriese AS, Philippe J, Van Renterghem DM et al., Carbamazepine hypersensitivity syndrome: report of 4 cases and review of the literature. *Medicine Baltimore* 1995; **74**:144–151.

10. Jones M, Fernandez Herrera J, Dorado JM et al., Epicutaneous test in carbamazepine cutaneous reactions. *Dermatology* 1994; **188**:18–20.

11. Küchler A, Hamm H, Weidenthaler-Barth B et al., Acute exanthematous pustulosis following oral nystatin therapy: a report of three cases. *Br J Dermatol* 1997; **137**:808–811.

12. Absar N, Daneshvar H, Beall G, Desensitization to trimethoprim/sulfamethoxazole in HIV-infected patients. *J Allergy Clin Immunol* 1994; **93**:1001–1005.

13. Belchi-Hernandez J, Espinosa-Parra FJ, Management of adverse reactions to prophylactic trimethoprim–sulfamethoxazole in patients with human immunodeficiency virus infection. *Ann Allergy Asthma Immunol* 1996; **76**:355–358.

14. Shapiro LE, Knowles SR, Shear NH, Comparative safety of tetracycline, minocycline, and doxycycline. *Arch Dermatol* 1997; **133**:1224–1230.

15. Klein GF, Kofler H, Wolf H, Fritsch PO, Eczema-like, erythematous, infiltrated plaques: a common side effect of subcutaneous heparin therapy. *J Am Acad Dermatol* 1989; **21**:703–707.

16. Rijlaarsdam U, Scheffer E, Meijer CJLM et al., Mycosis fungoides-like lesions associated with phenytoin and carbamazepine therapy. *J Am Acad Dermatol* 1991; **24**:216–220.

17. Bauer F, Quinacrine hydrochloride drug eruption (tropical lichenoid dermatitis). Its early and late sequelae and its malignant potential: a review. *J Am Acad Dermatol* 1981; **4**:239–248.

18. Shelley WB, Shelley ED, Talanin NY, Santoso-Pham J, Estrogen dermatitis. *J Am Acad Dermatol* 1995; **32**:25–31.

19. Hart R, Autoimmune progesterone dermatitis. *Arch Dermatol* 1977; **113**:426–430.

20. Stephens CJ, McFadden JP, Black MM, Rycroft RJ, Autoimmune progesterone dermatitis: absence of contact sensitivity to glucocorticoids, oestrogen and 17-alpha-OH-progesterone. *Contact Dermatitis* 1994; **31**:108–110.

21. Hogan DH, Maibach HI, Adverse dermatological reactions to transdermal drug delivery systems. *J Am Acad Dermatol* 1990; **22**:811–814.

22. Guin JD, Phillips D, Erythroderma from systemic contact dermatitis: a complication of systemic gentamicin in a patient with contact allergy to neomycin. *Cutis* 1989; **43**:564–567.

23. Breathnach SM, Mechanisms of drug eruptions: Part I. *Aust J Dermatol* 1995; **36**:121–127.

24. Troost RJ, Van Parys JA, Hooijkaas H et al., Allergy to carbamazepine: parallel in vivo and in vitro detection. *Epilepsia* 1996; **37**:1093–1099.

25. De Groot AC, *Patch testing*, 2nd edn. Amsterdam: Elsevier; 1994.

9. Contact Allergy Associated with Topical Treatment

Uwe Wollina

Topical treatment, although most widely used in dermatology, has had a renaissance in other medical fields. Some of the problems related to topical treatment in medicine are of importance in cosmetics and skin care too (see Chapters 12 and 13).

Antihistamines

Topically applied antihistamines may be classified according to their chemical nature (Table 9.1). In many cases, they can cause an irritant contact dermatitis (ICD). However, allergic contact sensitization has been documented as well.[1,2] Starting in the late 1940s, several reports appeared that described allergic contact dermatitis (ACD) to N-linked ethylene diamine derivatives such as tripelenamine, phenylpyramin and antazoline. Not only ointments but also eyedrops have been identified as a cause of allergic skin reactions. Cross reactions have been described in several but not all of these patients.[3] Allergic skin reactions and positive patch test reactions against O-linked ethanolamine derivatives such as diphenhydramine have been described in several papers. It is remarkable, that in some cases, the patch test results were negative on intact but became positive on stripped skin.[4]

Among the C-linked propylamine derivatives, chlorpheniramine maleate-containing eyedrops and creams have been shown to be responsible for chronic facial ACD.[5] Tripoline, initially developed for topical application, was withdrawn because of its allergic and irritant potential.

Phenothiazine derivatives were identified as inducers of ACD in the late 1950s, including promethazine, chlorpromazine and doxepin.[6] Adverse skin reactions to other antihistamines have been reported occasionally, e.g. piperazine

Table 9.1 Classification of antihistamines used topically
N-linked ethylene diamine derivatives
O-linked ethanolamine derivatives
C-linked propylamine derivatives
Phenothiazine derivatives
Others

dermatitis after accidental skin exposure[7] or occupational dermatitis to intermediates of H2-antagonists.[8]

The potency of topically applied antihistamines to cause skin irritancy and allergic dermatitis has to be recognized. In many countries, these drugs are available as over-the-counter (OTC) products. Their use in atopic dermatitis (AD) cannot be recommended.

Antimycotics

Topical antifungal substances are widely used and many of them are available as OTC products. Despite this fact and despite the irritant potential of some formulations, allergic contact reactions are rarely seen.

Imidazole derivatives have been reported to cause ACD.[9] Baes[10] reported a patient with ACD from miconazole. Patch testing with miconazole and other azole antimycotics revealed crossreactivity to compounds with β-substituted 1-phenethyl imidazoles showing an ortho-chlorine substitution of the aromatic ring, i.e. isoconazole, tioconazole, oxiconazole. Baes designed the name "ortho-chloro cross sensitivity" for this type of cross reaction.

In a Japanese study of 218 patch-tested patients with topical antimycotics, 18 were reactive showing 66 allergic reactions; 35 of these reactions were due to the antimycotic drug itself, and the others were contributed to emulsifiers, preservatives, etc. Allergic patch test reactions were observed to sulconazole (n = 16), croconazole (11), tioconazole (3), miconazole (3), bifonazole (1) and clotrimazole (1). Croconazole was rated the compound with the highest sensitizing potential, because significant shorter duration of treatment and smaller quantities of formulations were necessary to induce ACD, compared with other imidazole compounds.[11]

An unusual allergic skin eruption has been described in one women using topical isoconazole nitrate. She developed a papulopustular rash and a positive patch test reaction to 0.5% isoconazole nitrate. No cross reactions to other imidazoles were noted.[12]

Emulsifiers, additives and vehicles

Emulsifiers, additives and vehicles used in topical treatment can also be found in cosmetics and skin care products. In an Italian survey of 737 patients with suspected medicament- or cosmetic-related contact dermatitis, 39 (5.3%) gave positive patch test results to emulsifiers; 23 reactions were identified as clinically relevant, with triethanolamine as the most frequent sensitizer.[3]

In a recent study performed by the "Information Network of Dermatological Clinics (IVDK)" the authors suggested that allergic reactions to emulsifiers, additives and vehicles are not as frequent. In many cases it is the active ingredients that accompany these which are responsible for the adverse skin reactions. Among 2159 patients patch tested, only four of 14 substances tested had a frequency of allergic reaction higher than 1%: stearyl alcohol, cetylstearyl alcohol, tert-butylhydroquinone (a preservative) and lanolin. Patients at risk are those with atopic dermatitis or leg dermatitis (stasis dermatitis) and of older age.[14]

Allergic reactions against lanolin have been attributed to impurities but not to the lanolin itself. Use of purified lanolin preparations may lower the risk of unwanted side-effects of this excellent emulsifier. Patients with leg ulcers or stasis dermatitis are at risk. In 1410 patients tested, 262 positive allergic reactions have been documented (18.6%), which is about six times higher than in the average population.[15]

Preservatives

Medical preservatives are used in topical formulations worldwide. Individual prescriptions lacking in preservatives may be appropriate for highly sensitized patients. Kathon CG (Figure 9.1 and 9.2), parabens, propylene glycol, and formaldehyde are well known for their potential for allergic skin reactions and

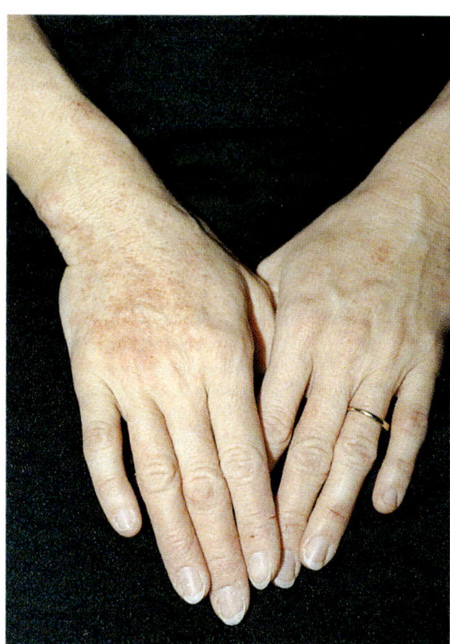

Figure 9.1: Allergic contact dermatitis to Kathon CG.

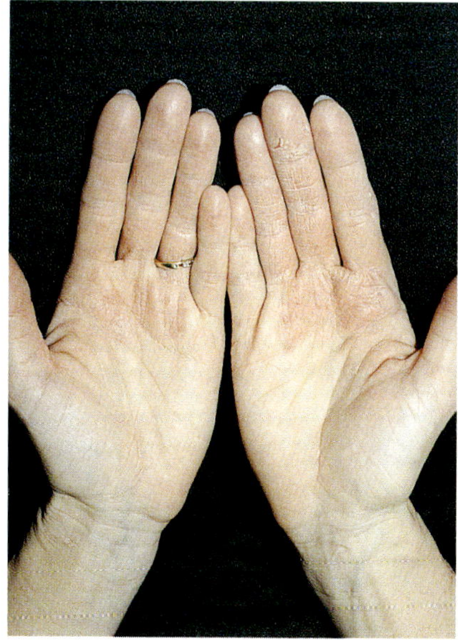

Figure 9.2: Allergic contact dermatitis to Kathon CG.

Table 9.2 Most common patch test reactions to preservatives in Germany[20]

Substance	*Test concentration (%)*	*Frequency of positive reactions (%)*
Thiomerosal	0.05	2.73
Benzalkonium chloride	0.1*	1.80
Chloracetamide	0.2	1.76
Phenyl mercuric acetate	100 ppm	1.42
Diazolidinyl urea	2	1.31
Dibromodicyanobutane/2-phenoxyethanol	0.5	1.20
Bronopol	0.5	1.02
Dibromo-dicyanobutane	0.1	1.02

*The concentration seems to be to high, since a significant number of irritant patch test reactions have been seen.

positive patch test reactions.[16,17] Formaldehyde sometimes but not always shows cross reactions to glutaraldehyde, which has been used as an antifungal agent to treat warts and hyperhidrosis.[18]

Propylene glycol has been assumed to cause not only ACD but also ICD and contact urticaria.[19] It is used in ointments and emollients and in medical lubricants. In a retrospective investigation of the IVDK, 2059 patients with more than 40,000 patch test reactions have been enrolled. In this large series only 1.08% of patients reacted to at least one substance.[20] The most common allergens are shown in Table 9.2.

Antipsoriatics

Salicylic acid is used in psoriasis treatment to remove the scales and support penetration of other antipsoriatic compounds. Moreover, it is widely used as a preservative. Although it is a rare sensitizer, it may be toxic if used under occlusion.[19] Anthralin (dithranol) is widely used in topical medications for psoriasis. It is known as a strong irritant but may sensitize occasionally.[21]

Ichthyol® (bitumen) and coal tar are antiproliferative and anti-inflammatory substances, that are known to sensitize skin against UV light. However, ACD is very rare.[19,22] Furocoumarins are used in photochemotherapy (PUVA). If applied topically, they are well known for phototoxic effects. Allergic contact sensitization has rarely been observed.[23]

Topical applied tazarotene, a newly developed receptor-selective retinoid, usually has mild irritant potential but ACD has not been reported yet.[24,25] For other antipsoriatics see the discussion of vitamins and related compounds later in this chapter.

Non-steroidal anti-inflammatory drugs (NSAIDs)

The domain of NSAIDs is the treatment of inflammatory joint and bone diseases. Their topical use is rather limited compared with the use of oral administration. However, there are several OTC products on the European market. ACD has been reported due to pyrazolones, propionic acid, indomethacin, bufexamac, piroxicam and different fenamates. Bufexamac dermatitis has been observed in patients with AD, with an incidence of about 0.1%. Among the arylpropionic acid derivatives, ketoprofen most frequently induces allergic reactions. About one half of them are photoallergic reactions. ACD has also been observed in topical treatment with ibuprofen, ibuproxan and oxyphenbutazon. Rare contact allergens are diclofenac, phenylbutazon and fenpradinol. An alternative NSAID is etofenamate, with which ACD and contact urticaria are very uncommon. As cross reactions among the different classes of the NSAIDs are not a major problem, treatment does not have to be discontinued if one NSAID can be replaced by another one.[26–28]

Scabicides

Benzoyl benzoate (30%) is used to treat scabies; ACD has not been reported but the induction of a pemphigoid bullous reaction has been observed in one patient. Crotamiton is used as a scabicide and antipruritic. It is a rare sensitizer, but patients with leg ulcers may be at risk. Gamma benzene hexachloride (Lindane) is used for scabies and pediculosis and may be toxic but allergic reactions have not been reported.[19] Permethrin, a synthetic pyrethroid, is probably the most effective topical treatment for scabies and may occasionally be a cause of ICD.[29,30]

Vitamins and related compounds

Retinoic acid, a derivative of vitamin A, causes an irritant dermatitis but exceptional cases with ACD have been reported.[19]

Hypersensitivity to thiamine (vitamin B1) probably accounts for the largest number of reported cutaneous side-effects to vitamins. Sensitization has been seen in exposed workers.

Dexpanthenol is closely related to the vitamin B complex. It is supposed to have wound-healing and revitalizing effects. It is also used in cosmetics (see Chapter 14). Unwanted side-effects are rare. Recently, a total of 40 cases from world literature have been reviewed. Patients with leg ulcers or stasis dermatitis in particular may develop ACD. Cross or group allergies have not been documented.[31]

Topical vitamin D derivatives such as tacalcitol and calcipotriol are currently widely used in psoriasis and other chronic inflammatory dermatoses. The creams and ointments may have some irritant potential, but allergic reactions are exceptional.[32]

Vitamin E is an antioxidant also used in burn care. When applied to skin, it may rarely lead to ICD and contact urticaria.[19]

Corticosteroids

Topical corticosteroids are among the most widely used drugs. In several countries, OTC products are available. Although side-effects are not uncommon, ACD has been observed in a number of cases.

In many cases, it is the preservatives and vehicles that are responsible for unwanted side-effects. Nevertheless, allergic reactions to topical hydrocortisone, tixocortol pivalate, prednisolone and prednicarbate, among others, have been reported in some patients (Figures 9.3 and 9.4).[33] Sensitization may occur due to topical application on skin or mucous membranes (e.g. nasal spray), and in some cases the reaction is boosted by oral or intravenous application. Budesonide, hydrocortisone-17-butyrate and tixocortol may be used as screening substances in patch series.[19,34] There is some crossreactivity between different corticosteroids, in particular between those of the hydrocortisone, triamcinolone and hydrocortisone-17-butyrate type.

The Leuven group in Belgium reported a prevalence of contact allergy to corticosteroids of up to 4.8% of tested patients.[35] Similar high frequencies have been reported from Finland[36] and England.[37]

In a German multicentre study, 1388 patients with suspected contact allergy against corticosteroids have been patch tested. In 1.1% a clinical relevant cutaneous sensitization against corticosteroids has been proved. The most common allergens were amcinonide, clobetasole propionate and hydrocortisone-17-butyrate.[38] One explanation for the relatively low frequency of corticosteroid allergies in this study may be that OTC products containing corticosteroids have not been on the German market, in contrast to several other countries. Lauerma[39] reported that corticosteroids of the betamethasone type (betamethasone and its disodium phosphate, dexamethasone, flucortolone and desoxymethasone) are the least common allergens in Finland.

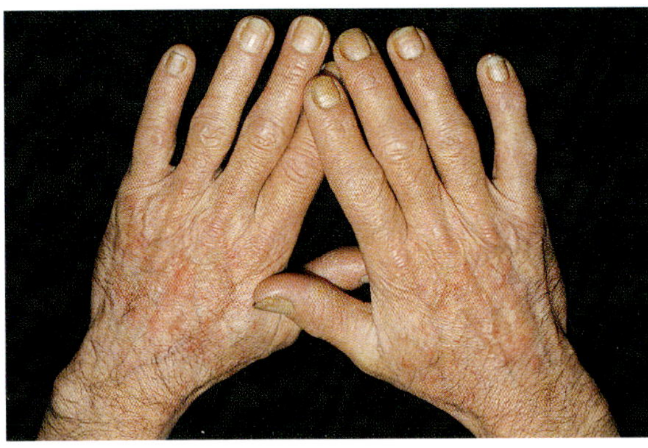

Figure 9.3: Allergic contact dermatitis to a chloroxylenol-containing cream.

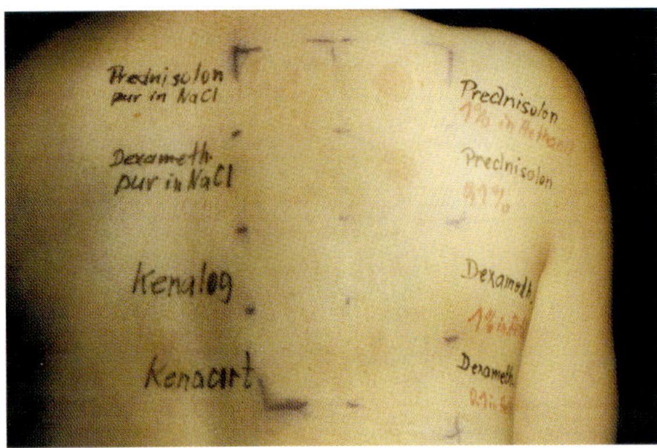

Figure 9.4: Positive patch test reaction to prednisolone.

Corticosteroid allergy may be a clue to reactivity against other endogenous hormones including adrenocorticotrophic hormone (ACTH) or progesterone.[19]

Wound-care products

It is not completely understood why patients with chronic venous insufficiency are prone to develop cutaneous side-effects, but damage to perilesional skin barrier function in leg ulcer patients seems to be a major factor.

Topical antibiotics are still used in the treatment of chronic wounds, though they may cause a delay of wound healing and ACD. Neomycin, framycetin, and chloramphenicol are among the most common allergens in patients with leg ulcers or stasis dermatitis.[40,41] Sensitization may also develop during the use of ophthalmological topical products. Zaki et al.[42] noted a higher frequency of positive patch test results to bacitracin in 85 patients with leg ulcers.

Nowadays, as complementary medicine has gained popularity, the frequency of allergic reactions to propolis has increased and accounted for 9.2% in 811 patients tested for stasis dermatitis.[40]

Balsam of Peru has been used for many years to improve granulation in chronic and burn wounds. As it is a common ingredient of skin-care products and anal therapeutics, sensitization is not uncommon; figures obtained are 24% in 101 children, 6% in 2000 adults[43] and 19.3% in adult patients with stasis dermatitis.[40] Cross reactions are based on ingredients such as cinnamic acid and aldehyde which both Balsam of Peru and fragrances have in common. Therefore, not all sensitization is caused by topical treatment, sometimes it is caused by cosmetic intolerance.

Modern hydrocolloid or hydrogel dressings bear an exceptional low risk of ACD and can, therefore, be recommended for the highly sensitized patients. Problems may arise from colophonyrosin in some of the hydrocolloid dressings. Helland et al.[44] reported on ACD in two patients whose leg ulcers were covered with Synthaderm. Patch tests were negative to isothiocyanates isolated from the dressing but positive to Synthaderm samples. ACD has not been reported for hydropolymers or alginates.

Products using acrylate glues should be avoided in acrylate sensitized patients.[45,46]

Transdermal treatment systems (TTS)

These have been developed for topical application but systemic delivery of different drugs. Skin irritation has been observed in about 15% of patients using nitroglycerine TTS. Allergic reactions have been reported in up to 50% for clonidine TTS and pyridostimine bromide TTS. About 7% of nicotine TTS users and up to 17% of patients treated with oestradiol TTS experience some unwanted side-effects but, as in other cases of TTS, most often it is the glues, components of the matrix or penetration enhancers that are responsible. Only a minor number are of an allergic nature.[47,48]

References

1. Fisher AA, The antihistamines. *J Am Acad Dermatol* 1980; **3**:303–306.
2. Szolar-Platzer C, Maibach HI, Allergic contact dermatitis to topically applied antihistamines. *Derm Beruf Umwelt* 1996; **44**:205–212.
3. Epstein E, Allergy to dermatologic agents. *JAMA* 1966; **198**:517–520.
4. Vickers CFH, Dermatitis medicamentosa. *Br Med J* 1961; **1**:1366–1367.

5. Tosti A, Bardazzi F, Pincastelli E, Contact dermatitis due to chlorpheniramine maleate in eyedrops. *Contact Dermatitis* 1990; **22**:55.

6. Ippen H, Berufsbedingte Hautveränderungen durch Phenothiazin-Derivate. *Derm Beruf Umwelt* 1959; **7**:12–21.

7. Calnan CD, Occupational piperazine dermatitis. *Contact Dermatitis* 1975; **2**:126.

8. Rycroft RJG, Allergic contact dermatitis from a novel diamino intermediate, 5-[(2-aminoethyl)thiomethyl-*N,N*-dimethyl-2-furan] methanamine, in laboratory synthesis. *Contact Dermatitis* 1983; **9**:456–458.

9. Guidetti MS, Vincenzi C, Guerra L, Tosti A, Contact dermatitis due to imidazole antimycotics. *Contact Dermatitis* 1995; **33**:282.

10. Baes H, Contact sensitivity to miconazole with ortho-chloro cross-sensitivity to other imidazoles. *Contact Dermatitis* 1991; **24**:89–93.

11. Yoneyama E, Allergic contact dermatitis due to topical imidazole antimycotics. The sensitizing ability of active ingredients and cross-sensitivity. *Nippon Ika Daigaku Zasshi* 1996; **63**:356–364.

12. Lazarov A, Ingber A, Pustular allergic contact dermatitis to isoconazole nitrate. *Am J Contact Dermatitis* 1997; **8**:229–230.

13. Tosti A, Guerra L, Morelli R, Bardazzi F, Prevalence and source of sensitization to emulsifiers: a clinical study. *Contact Dermatitis* 1990; **23**:68–72.

14. Schnuch A, Arnold R, Bahmer F et al., Epikutantestung mit der Salbengrundlagenreihe. Ergebnisse des “Informationsverbundes Dermatologischer Kliniken” (IVDK). *Derm Beruf Umwelt* 1993; **41**:176–183.

15. Nachbar F, Korting HC, Plewig G, Zur Bedeutung des positiven Epikutantests auf Lanolin. *Derm Beruf Umwelt* 1993; **41**:227–236.

16. De Groot AC, Weyland JW, Bos JD, Jagtmann BA, Contact allergy to preservatives (I). *Contact Dermatitis* 1986; **14**:120–121.

17. De Groot AC, Bos JD, Jagtmann BA et al., Contact allergy to preservatives (II). *Contact Dermatitis* 1986; **15**:218–222.

18. Jordan WP, Dahl MV, Albert HL, Contact dermatitis from glutaraldehyde. *Arch Dermatol* 1972; **105**:94–95.

19. Rietschel RL, Fowler Jr JF, *Fisher's Contact Dermatitis*, 4th edn. Baltimore: Williams & Wilkins; 1995.

20. Brasch J, Henseler T, Frosch P, Patch test reactions to a preliminary preservative series. A retrospective study based on data collected by the “Information Network of Dermatological Clinics” (IVDK) in Germany. *Derm Beruf Umwelt* 1993; **41**:71–76.

21. De Groot AC, Nater JP, Contact allergy to dithranol. *Contact Dermatitis* 1981; **7**:5–8.

22. Wollina U, Hein G, Knopf B. *Psoriasis und Gelenkerkrankungen: Pathogenese, Klinik, Diagnostik, Therapie*. Jena: Gustav Fischer Verlag; 1996.

23. Plewig G, Hofmann C, Braun-Falco O, Photoallergic dermatitis from 8-methoxy psoralen. *Arch Dermatol Res* 1978; **261**:201–211.

24. Marks R, Clinical safety of tazarotene in the treatment of plaque psoriasis. *J Am Acad Dermatol* 1997; **37**:S25–S32.

25. Wollina U, Genital ulcers in a psoriasis patient using topical tazarotene. *Br J Dermatol* 1998; **138**:713–14.

26. Gebhardt M, Reuter A, Knopf B, Allergic contact dermatitis from topical diclofenac. *Contact Dermatitis* 1994; **30**:183–184.

27. Gebhardt M, Wollina U, Kutane Nebenwirkungen nichtsteroidaler Antiphologistika (NSAID). *Z Rheumatol* 1995; **54**:405–412.

28. Ophaswongse S, Maibach H, Topical nonsteroidal antiinflammatory drugs: allergic and photoallergic contact dermatitis and phototoxicity. *Contact Dermatitis* 1993; **29**:57–64.

29. Elgart ML, A risk–benefit assessment of agents used in the treatment of scabies. *Drug Safety* 1996; **14**:386–393.

30. Flannigan SA, Tucker SB, Key MM et al., Primary irritant contact dermatitis from synthetic pyrethroid insecticide exposure. *Arch Toxicol* 1985; **56**:288–294.

31. Schmid-Grendelmeier P, Wyss M, Elsner P, Contact allergy to dexpanthenol. A report of seven cases and review of the literature. *Derm Beruf Umwelt* 1995; **43**:175–178.

32. Yip J, Goodfield M, Contact dermatitis from MC 903, a topical vitamin D3 analog. *Contact Dermatitis* 1991; **25**:139–140.

33. Dunkel FG, Elsner P, Burg G, Allergic contact dermatitis from prednicarbate. *Contact Dermatitis* 1991; **24**:59–60.

34. Lauerma AI, Reitamo S, Maibach HI, Systemic hydrocortisone/cortisol induces allergic skin reactions in presensitized subjects. *J Am Acad Dermatol* 1991; **24**:182–185.

35. Dooms-Goosens, Degreef HJ, Marien KJ et al., Contact allergy to corticosteroids. A frequently missed diagnosis. *J Am Acad Dermatol* 1989; **21**:538–543.

36. Lauerma AI, Reitamo S, Contact allergy to corticosteroids. *J Am Acad Dermatol* 1993; **28**:618–622.

37. Wilkinson SM, Cartwright PH, English JSC, Hydrocortisone: an important cutaneous allergen. *Lancet* 1991; **337**:761–762.

38. Lehmann P, Aberer W, Bäurle G et al., Corticosteroid contact dermatitis. Results of a multicenter study from the German Contact Dermatitis Group. *Derm Beruf Umwelt* 1997; **45**:116–120.

39. Lauerma AI, Screening for corticosteroid contact sensitivity. Comparision of tixocortol pivalate, hydrocortinsone-17-butyrate and hydrocortisone. *Contact Dermatitis* 1991; **24**:123–130.

40. Lange-Ionescu S, Pilz B, Geier J, Frosch PJ, Kontaktallergien bei Patienten mit Stauungsdermatitis oder Ekzem der Beine. Ergebnisse des Informationsverbunds Dermatologischer Kliniken und der Deutschen Kontaktallergiegruppe. *Derm Beruf Umwelt* 1996; **44**:14–22.

41. Paramsothy Y, Collins M, Smith GA, Contact dermatitis in patients with leg ulcers. *Contact Dermatitis* 1988; **18**:30–36.

42. Zaki I, Shall L, Dalziel KL, Bacitracin: a significant sensitizer in ulcer patients? *Contact Dermatitis* 1994; **31**:92–94.

43. Fregert S, Möller H, Contact allergy to balsam of Peru. *Br J Dermatol* 1963; **75**:218–222.

44. Helland S, Nyfors A, Utne L, Contact dermatitis to Synthaderm. *Contact Dermatitis* 1983; **9**:504–506.

45. Wollina U, Moderne Wunddressings – ein Update. *Vasomed* 1997; **9**:148–152.

46. Wollina U, Lokaltherapie chronischer Wunden mit einem neuen Hydropolymerverband – klinische Erfahrungen bei 478 Patienten. *Z Hautkrankh* 1997; **72**:500–506.

47. Wollina U, Transdermale therapeutische Systeme (TTS) – Übersicht zu Techniken, Wirkstoffen, Indikationen und Nebenwirkungen. *Med Welt* 1991; **42**:877–880.

48. Hogan DJ, Maibach HI, Adverse dermatologic reactions to transdermal drug delivery formulations. *J Am Acad Dermatol* 1990; **22**:811–814.

10. Occupational Contact Dermatitis

Health Professions

Matthias Gebhardt

Occupational skin disease in health professions have been well known for more than a century. When the Hungarian I. Semmelweis introduced chloric calcium as the first hand antiseptic in obstetrics he thereby saved hundreds of lives of mothers giving birth. However, a large number of reactions to this strong irritant occurred among nurses, midwifes and obstetricians. Many irritants are still present in medicine. Among them, wet work conditions is top of the list, along with skin occlusion due to gloves, contact with disinfectants, the need for intensive skin cleansing and some specific factors in particular fields of medicine.

Irritant contact dermatitis (ICD) is the most frequent diagnosis among all occupational skin diseases in health professionals. Allergic contact dermatitis (ACD) may develop subsequently, as a result of chronic skin irritation. Those employees exposed to wet work who have a history of atopic dermatitis or hand dermatitis are more susceptible to ICD. Once they acquire occupational contact dermatitis on their hands, they have a poorer prognosis than their non-atopic counterparts.[1] There is a close overlap among the causative triad ICD, ACD and atopic skin/atopic dermatitis (AD). Most individuals affected by ACD also suffer from skin irritation. ICD is frequently associated with a history of AD or current atopic skin disease. Therefore, it makes no sense to look separately for ACD, ICD and AD in health professionals. For medicolegal reasons it is, however, important to distinguish between job-related ICD or ACD, and ICD based on the natural course of a pre-existing AD.

Studies on ICD in women show that the worst prognosis is associated with continuing irritant exposure at home (household work, child care, etc.). Domestic exposure hazards are especially relevant for healthcare professions, in which women are employed in a high percentage. Among physicians, however, the frequency of hand dermatitis is higher in men than in women, as shown in a Norwegian questionnaire survey.[2]

Looking at the distribution of skin disorders in various medical professions, it is not the physician who is most affected by ICD but technicians, radiology assistants, and hospital cleaning and kitchen workers.[2] In a questionnaire-based study, 33% of catering staff and 35% of women cleaners in a large hospital reported skin problems – hand dermatitis in 15% of the caterers and 12% of the cleaners.[3] In the majority, the dermatitis was irritant in origin and related to wet work occupations. So, with increasing professional status, the risk of developing skin disease decreases. Nevertheless, the rate of occupational skin disease in medicine is far too high, being highest in cleaners and hospital kitchen workers, less in hospital nurses and doctor's assistants and least in highly qualified physicians. Natural rubber latex gloves and disinfectants have been found to be the main causes of self-reported skin problems in health care.[4]

Gloves

Development of **contact allergy** is facilitated by irritation of the skin. This is one reason for the high percentage of contact allergies in the health care professions. From the dermatologist's point of view, probably the main allergic occupational health problem in these professions is allergy to natural rubber latex and rubber chemicals. Although this is extensively dealt with in other chapters of this book, it is worth focusing on a few aspects here. The use of rubber gloves has increased considerably during the last two decades due to improvement of preventive efforts. The awareness of the hazards of AIDS, different forms of infectious hepatitis and other infectious diseases, the increased number of patients treated in haemodialysis, transplantation and intensive care units, and the increasing number of aggressive antineoplastic treatments are just a few factors in the need for increased use of protective gloves by healthcare workers. Use of gloves has caused an dramatic increase of health problems. Table 10.1 lists possible skin disturbances attributed to rubber gloves.

Immediate-type allergy to natural rubber latex appears mainly as contact urticaria and/or mucosal allergy corresponding to the mode of sensitization (contact or aerogeneous). Although contact urticaria is caused by direct skin contact with latex gloves, it may spread to remote regions and even cause systemic symptoms. Risk factors for sensitization to latex include frequent use of disposable gloves, presence of prior atopic disease, prior or current hand dermatitis and surgical work.[5–7]

Glove powder may irritate skin areas covered by the glove and carries latex particles on its surface. Therefore it enhances the probability of acquiring immediate-type latex allergy – by the respiratory or skin route – and latex protein contact dermatitis. Irritated skin with damaged epidermal barrier function is also more likely to become allergic to rubber chemicals. Thus, avoiding powdered gloves, no matter what kind of powder is used, is a more certain way of preventing occupational skin disease in health professionals. There are comfortable alternatives, which have interior coatings that facilitate sliding the

Table 10.1 Manifestations of skin diseases caused by rubber gloves

- Local pruritus
- Contact urticaria
  - IgE-mediated (anaphylactic reaction is the maximal manifestation)
  - Non-immunological contact urticaria
- Contact dermatitis
  - Irritant contact dermatitis
  - Allergic contact dermatitis
  - Protein contact dermatitis
- Deterioration of pre-existing conditions
  - Atopic dermatitis
  - Various skin diseases (Koebner's phenomenon in psoriasis, lichen, etc.)

hands into non-powdered gloves, however these are usually more expensive. A cotton glove worn under a rubber glove can also improve the disease.

Occlusion by gloves contributes to their negative effects on the skin. The skin becomes moist and soft beneath the glove material and dries out very fast and becomes chapped after removing the gloves. Application of protective creams before glove use and skin-care creams and lotions after work are options to lower glove-induced skin damage.

When testing health professionals for occupational skin disease it is highly recommended that the test procedures for natural rubber latex (NRL) allergy, listed in Table 10.2, are included.

Disinfectants

Disinfectants such as formaldehyde are well known as irritants and allergens. Formaldehyde-based disinfectants were widely substituted in the 1970s and 1980s by glutaraldehyde. Unfortunately, the latter has taken over the role of formaldehyde in terms of hazardous skin effects. Glutaraldehyde and formaldehyde do not crossreact with each other.[9] Formaldehyde itself is still widely used in histology laboratories and, to a much lesser extent, in a few instrumental and surface disinfectants. Traces of formaldehyde are present in a wide range of objects such as paper towels, lotions and creams preserved by formaldehyde releasers, and in protective clothing; the allergic individual needs to be very highly sensitized in order to be affected by these low amounts of formaldehyde. Another disinfectant of increasing occupational relevance in medicine is glyoxal.[10] Exposure to these three disinfectant substances is most likely when disinfecting surfaces or instruments; they are almost never used in skin disinfection. For the latter, alcohol, which is less allergenic, is far more often used.

Table 10.2 Test procedures for NRL allergy (adapted from Maso and Goldberg[8])

Test		Indication
1. Prick test with saline in which the patient's own gloves have been incubated	→	Immediate-type reaction to latex?
2. Patch test with glove material (approximately 1 cm^2 piece) and rubber chemical series provided by several companies	→	Allergic contact dermatitis to glove material?
3. Scratch-chamber test with moistened glove material if (1) and (2) are negative	→	Protein contact dermatitis to latex protein?
4. 'Use' test with one glove finger on wet skin for 20 min	→	IgE-mediated urticaria (or non-immunological contact urticaria)?

Be prepared to treat anaphylaxis due to testing!

In patch testing disinfectants the problem is always finding the right test concentrations. There is a fine balance between test-induced skin irritation and missing a genuine allergic reaction due to over-dilution. So discussion of the right glutaraldehyde concentration continues. A German multicentre study demonstrated a high number of irritant and questionable reactions with the usual 1% pet formulation,[11] indicating too high a test concentration. For testing patient's own workplace disinfectants, I recommend using concentration ranges that start at the concentration the patient uses (or, to increase the safety of the test, 10% of this concentration, depending on the disinfectant) and diluting down to 1/100 of the highest concentration. Whenever a positive reaction is observed, 10 non-exposed controls should be tested along with the patient. Known allergenic ingredients should be tested separately in the recommended concentrations.

Mercury

Sensitization to inorganic mercury compounds may arise from liquid mercury released by broken thermometers. Topical disinfectants based on organic mercury compounds are still on the market. They should be avoided due to their allergenic properties and banned because of toxic effects (due to skin absorption).

One organic mercury compound, thimerosal (thiomersal, merthiolate) has particular relevance for medical professions. It is among the world's 10 most common contact allergens when routinely tested in a standard series.[12] Most health-care workers, physicians, laboratory technicians and other personnel employed in medicine are vaccinated against hepatitis, and most of the vaccines contain thimerosal as a preservative. Many individuals have been sensitized to thimerosal by these vaccinations without having had any complaints after receiving the injections, as I and others have shown previously.[13] Although some studies have proved good tolerance of thimerosal-containing vaccines in patients sensitized to this compound, general practitioners can have legal problems in giving the injections because of the attached notice to each container "not to use in patients allergic to any compound of this vaccine. . .". Alternative vaccines, free of thimerosal, are not available in most countries. This example highlights the difficulties that may arise when obtaining positive reactions that have no clinical relevance. I recommend not testing thimerosal in standard series, only including it when testing for allergy to topical eye preparations, where it may be present in eye lens storage liquids. Thimerosal may also be present in veterinary skin disinfectants. It is irritant in higher concentrations, therefore weak or questionable reactions should be regarded with caution.

Acrylic bone cement

Orthopaedic surgeons are at risk of acquiring contact allergy to acrylic bone cement. Based on methyl methacrylate, this agent is a common sensitizer among surgical specialities. Unfortunately, most surgical rubber gloves are easily penetrated within a minute or less by the acrylic monomer; even wearing two gloves on each hand is not very effective skin protection against the substance. Alternatives are PVP gloves consisting of an outer layer of polyethylene, an intermediary layer of ethylene vinyl alcohol copolymer and an inner layer of polyethylene, or the 4H (Safety 4, Denmark) glove which has found wide acceptance in occupational dermatology.[14,15]

Pharmaceuticals

Pharmaceuticals dissolved by injecting diluents into the drug container or drug preparations drawn into syringes from vials are frequently spilled on the hands of the nurse or doctor preparing the injection or infusion, because of the vacuum or overpressure arising during the procedure. This was once one of the major ways of acquiring an allergy to injectable drugs such as antibiotics. Today, pressure compensation valves between the vial and the syringe are common measures used to prevent spillage of medicaments onto unprotected skin. Skin contact with tablets can also cause sensitization or elicitation of contact dermatitis. Nevertheless, both these modes of sensitization still exist.

It is likely that there are more cases than are detected. Difficulties in investigation for the causative drug contribute to this. It takes attentive observation of the affected person and repeated observation of the course of a given skin disease to identify the triggers, because many hundreds of different contacts occur each day. Of course, it is easier to screen with a rubber series or test half a dozen disinfectants than to include the many different pharmaceuticals in the patch test. Sometimes, changing departments may give additional evidence of a particular cause, when a nurse or doctor is affected (e.g. leaving psychiatry for orthopaedics means avoiding psychopharmaceuticals as a possible cause of skin complaints, etc.).

Drugs commonly involved in ACD are antibiotics, psychiatric drugs and sedatives, local anaesthetics, antihypertensive drugs, hormones and several other classes of agents.

Special problems arise with antineoplastic drugs. Skin irritation among medical personnel is commonly observed when exposing unprotected skin.[16] For patch tests it is very difficult to find the right test concentrations. Testing controls is also not easily done because skin absorption of these agents may cause mutagenous and teratogenous effects. De Groot[17] gives test concentrations for some agents in his book. Avoidance and re-introduction in the workplace may prove the relevance of questionable test reactions.

Veterinary professions

Veterinary surgeons are exposed to almost the same group of allergens and irritants as doctors, but there are some additional ones. Protein contact dermatitis due to animal proteins has been reported following exposure of obstetric veterinarians to bovine amniotic fluid. A scratch-chamber test with these fluids can be done to exclude their causative role. Many other animal proteins should be considered as protein contact allergens. In a statistical survey of Finland

Table 10.3 Antibiotics reported to have caused occupational allergies in veterinary medicine

Furazolidone
Neomycin
Olaquindox
Penethamate BP
Penicillin
Spiramycin
Streptomycin
Tylosin

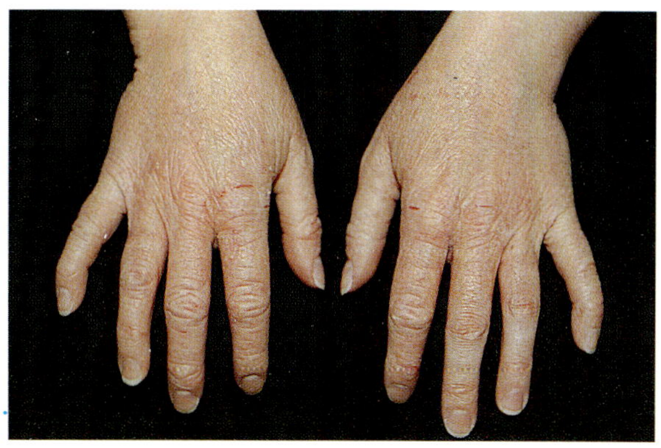

Figure 10.1: Irritative hand eczema in a nurse.

veterinarians ranked fourth (per 100,000 employees) in terms of occupational contact urticaria and protein contact dermatitis.[18] In the same study physicians were eleventh, dentists and nurses fourteenth and fifteenth. These data show the special importance of IgE-mediated skin diseases in veterinarians.

Because infections and infestations are a major problem in veterinary medicine, antiparasitics (carbamates, pyrethroids, etc.) are important drug allergens. The same is true of fungicides. Balsam of Peru is used by some farmers to treat ectoparasites in cattle. There many case reports, and Hjorth et al.[19] have shown antibiotics (Table 10.3) to be of occupational relevance. Many antibiotics are still used in cattle breeding in order to improve the disease resistance of the animals. The photoallergenic agent olaquindox has been added in relevant concentrations to mineral feed (1000mg/kg) and prefabricated fodder (50mg/kg).[20,21] However, this is more important for veterinary assistants and cattle breeders than for the veterinary surgeons themselves. When testing a veterinarian, it is always best to ask her or him to bring the most used pharmaceuticals for the test and not to rely on test-tray recommendations.

References

1. Nilsson E, Back O, The importance of anamnestic information of atopy, metal dermatitis and earlier hand eczema for the development of hand dermatitis in women in wet hospital work. *Acta Derm Venereol (Stockh)* 1986; **66**:45–50.

2. Kavli G, Angell E, Moseng D, Hospital employees and skin problems. *Contact Dermatitis* 1987; **17**:156–158.

3. Gawkrodger DJ, Lloyd MH, Hunter JA, Occupational skin disease in hospital cleaning and kitchen workers. *Contact Dermatitis* 1986; **15**:132–135.

4. Stingeni L, Lapomarda V, Lisi P, Occupational hand dermatitis in hospital environments. *Contact Dermatitis* 1995; **33**:172–176.

5. Hunt LW, Fransway AF, Reed CE et al., An epidemic of occupational allergy to latex involving health care workers. *J Occup Environ Med* 1995; **37**:1204–1209.

6. Field EA, Atopy and other risk factors for UK dentists reporting an adverse reaction to latex gloves. *Contact Dermatitis* 1998; **38**:132–136.

7. Turjanmaa K, Incidence of immediate allergy to latex gloves in hospital personnel. *Contact Dermatitis* 1987; **17**:270–275.

8. Maso MJ, Goldberg DJ, Contact dermatoses from disposable glove use: a review. *J Am Acad Dermatol* 1990; **23**:733–737.

9. Maibach HI, Glutaraldehyde: cross reactions to formaldehyde. *Contact Dermatitis* 1975; **1**:326–327.

10. Elsner P, Pevny I, Burg G, Occupational contact dermatitis due to glyoxal in health care workers. *Am J Contact Dermatitis* 1990; **1**:250–253.

11. Schnuch A, Geier J, Glutardialdehyd – Berufsspektrum eines Allergens. *Dermatosen* 1995; **43**:30–31.

12. Storrs FJ, Rosenthal LE, Adams RM et al., Prevalence and relevance of allergic reactions in patients patch tested in North America – 1984 to 1985. *J Am Acad Dermatol* 1989; **20**:1038–1045.

13. Gebhardt M, Zur Relevanz der positiven Epikutantestreaktion auf Thiomersal. *Dermatosen* 1995; **43**:122–125.

14. Darre E, Vedel P, Jensen JS, Skin protection against methylmethacrylate. *Acta Orthop Scand* 1987; **58**:236–238.

15. Tobler M, Freiburghaus AU, A glove with exceptional protective features minimizes the risks of working with hazardous chemicals. *Contact Dermatitis* 1992; **26**:299–303.

16. Fisher AA, Allergic contact reactions in health personnel. *J Allergy Clin Immunol* 1992; **90**:729–738.

17. De Groot AC, *Patch testing*, 2nd edn. Amsterdam: Elsevier; 1994.

18. Kanerva L, Toikkanen J, Jolanki R, Estlander T, Statistical data on occupational contact urticaria. *Contact Dermatitis* 1996; **35**:229–233.

19. Hjorth N, Roed-Petersen J, Allergic contact dermatitis in veterinary surgeons. *Contact Dermatitis* 1980; **6**:27–29.

20. Schauder S, The dangers of olaquindox. Photoallergy, chronic photosensitive dermatitis and extreme increased photosensitivity in the human, hypoaldosteronism in swine. *Dermatosen* 1989; **37**:183–185.

21. Schauder S, Schröder W, Geier J, Olaquindox-induced airborne photoallergic contact dermatitis followed by transient or persistent light reactions in 15 pig breeders. *Contact Dermatitis* 1996; **35**:344–354.

METALWORKERS

Undine Berndt

The profession of a metalworker includes various processes, with the major aim of shaping raw metal pieces into finished products such as instruments, tools and machine components, mainly by using machine techniques. Although simple tools and manually operated machines have been supplemented or replaced by semi- or fully automatic ones, the metalworking industry is a trade that still involves a lot of work by hand. Consequently, the parts of the body which are predominantly affected by occupational skin disease are the hands and forearms. As epidemiological data from insurance companies shows, irritant as well as allergic contact dermatitis (ACD) is a common finding in metalworkers[1,2] and forms the main proportion of occupational skin diseases in this profession.

What causes contact dermatitis in this profession?

Irritants

Preparation of the raw material as well as the finishing touches often require manual work at the workbench using hand tools, such as files and scrapers, which naturally involves friction and pressure on the worker's hands. After adjusting the piece being worked and the machine a hardened tool edge removes chips by different mechanical means, such as turning, drilling, grinding, shaping and planing. All these processes have in common the fact that most of the invested energy is transformed into heat due to surface friction and plastic deformation of the metal.[3] This heat can damage both the machine and the work piece. It is therefore necessary to use cutting fluids, which carry away produced heat and decrease its production by lubricating the area between the tool and the metal to minimize friction.[4,5] Depending on the cutting operation and the raw material, two different major types of cutting fluids are used: mineral oil lubricants (neat oils) and water-miscible coolants. The latter are complex mixtures that include emulsifiers, extreme pressure additives, corrosion inhibitors, coupling agents, stabilizers, biocides, antifoam agents, dyes and fragrances together with (soluble oils) or without (synthetic fluids) mineral oils.[6] By handling the work piece and operating the machines, machinists are frequently or even permanently exposed to cutting fluids, which are considered to be the most important skin hazard in this occupation. During the first half of the twentieth century the most common cutaneous problem of machinists using neat oils was oil acne; nowadays, with the increasing use of mainly water-based metalworking fluids, eczematous contact dermatitis has become the most common skin disease in these workers.[4] The alkaline pH of the cooling agents, which can increase further due to concentration of the fluid in use, irritates the skin of hands and forearms.[7,8] Additionally, metal shavings may cause microtraumata that allow chemical irritants and allergens to enter the skin easier. After finishing the process, machines must be regularly maintained and lubricated. Swarf is removed from the working zone. Solvents are used to clean mineral oils from processed metal products and skin.

Allergens

Various constituents of the cutting fluids are potential sensitizers leading to allergic reactions, especially on already irritated skin. Some of them release formaldehyde, which is also a common allergen, and biocides such as chlormethylisothiazolone (Kathon CG) are common allergens in cutting fluids, too (See Figure 10.2).

Metals, such as nickel, cobalt, and potassium dichromate are also an important cause of ACD in machinists as well.[9] They may be liberated in fluids during the cutting procedure, reaching significant concentrations.

Endogenic predisposition factor

There is a quantity of published data indicating that subjects with an atopic skin diathesis are more prone to develop hand eczema than those without this disposition.[10–12]

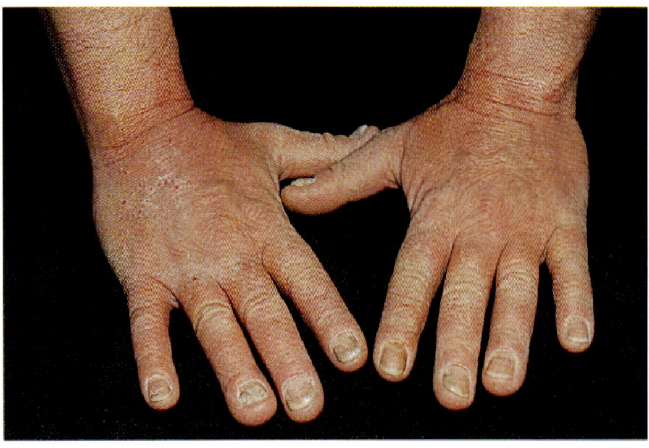

Figure 10.2: The hands of a machinist show allergic contact dermatitis to biocides in metal-working fluid.

Table 10.4 Specific screening patch tests for metal workers*

Allergen (trade name)	*Concentration and vehicle*	*Function*
1-Aza-5-ethyl-3,7-dioxabicyclo(3,3,0)octane (Bioban CS 1246)†	1% pet	Biocide, formaldehyde releaser
p-Chloro-m-xylenol	1% pet	Biocide, coupling agent
2-Bromo-2-nitro-1,3-propandiole (Bronopol)	0.5% pet	Biocide, formaldehyde releaser
Chloroacetamide	0.2% pet	Biocide
1,3,5-Tris(2-hydroxyethyl)-hexahydrotriazine (Grotan BK)	1% pet	Biocide, formaldehyde releaser
4-Aminoazobenzol (Solvent Yellow 1)	1% pet	Colour
Triclosan (Irgasan DP 300)	2% pet	Biocide
Benzotriazole	1% pet	Corrosion inhibitor
Benzylhemiformal (Preventol D2)	1% pet	Biocide, formaldehyde releaser
p-tert-Butylcatechin	1% pet	
Triethanolamine	2.5% pet	Emulsifier, corrosion inhibitor
Lanolin alcohol (Amerchol L101)	50% pet	Emulsifier, emollient
Dipentene	2% pet	Extreme pressure additive, fragrance
Dichlorophene	0.5% pet	Biocide
Monoethanolamine	2% pet	Emulsifier, corrosion inhibitor
Abietic acid	10% pet	Main component of colophony, emulsifier
Diethanolamine	2% pet	Corrosion inhibitor
2-Hydroxymethyl-2-nitro-1,3-propandiol (Tris Nitro)†	1% pet	Biocide, formaldehyde releaser
4,4-Dimethyloxazolidine + 3,4,4-trimethyloxazolidine (Bioban CS 1135)	1% pet	Biocide, formaldehyde releaser
4-(2-Nitrobutyl)morpholine + 4,4'-(2-ethyl-2-nitrotrimethylene)-dimorpholine (Bioban P 1487)†	1% pet	Biocide, formaldehyde releaser
Coconut diethanolamide (Comperlan KD)	0.5% pet	Emulsifier, foam stabilizer
2-n-Octyl-4-isothiazolin-3-one (Kathon 893)	0.025% pet	Biocide
Cl-Methylisothiazolone (Kathon CG)	0.01% aq	Biocide
Methylene-bis-oxazolidine (Grotan OD)	1% pet	Biocide, formaldehyde releaser
Dibromodicyanobutane (Tektamer 38, Euxyl K 400)	0.3% pet	Biocide
1,2-Benzisothiazolin-3-one (Proxel)	0.1% pet	Biocide

*Common additives to metal-working fluids and their function (metal-working industry/technical fluids patch test series adapted from HERMAL according to advice of the German Contact Allergy Group (DKG) and Information Network of Dermatological Clinics (IVDK).[13]
†Use in metal-working fluids forbidden in Germany.[14]

Diagnosis

When hand eczema has been diagnosed, a very careful investigation of the causative factor(s) should follow. Therefore a detailed history of occupation and domestic exposures, and their possible relationship to the occurrence of skin damage, is necessary. In the case of a suspected allergy, standard and specific screening patch test series should be performed (Table 10.4). Apart from this, it is recommended that one tests non-irritant dilutions of the involved substances, such as fresh and used metalworking fluids, barrier creams and soaps, as well as their components.

How can contact dermatitis be prevented?

In order to avoid skin irritation it is essential to reduce skin contact to potential irritants as far as possible. Protective gloves are generally considered a safety hazard and should not be worn during the cutting process because they increase the danger of severe accidents if they become entangled in moving parts.[4] They should be used when handling aggressive solvents and degreasers. Frequent cleaning of hands with mild detergents and regular use of skin-care products and barrier creams are recommended, but even these substances as well as frequent water contact may cause irritation, and additives in creams and soaps may be sensitizers. Atopics especially should be thoroughly informed about their increased risk of becoming affected by hand eczema and about preventive measures to avoid its occurrence.

References

1. Diepgen TL, Schmidt A, Schmidt M, Fartasch M, Demographic and legal characteristics of occupational skin diseases. *Allergologie* 1994; **17**:84–89.

2. Goh CL, Gan SL, The incidence of cutting fluid dermatitis among metalworkers in a metal fabrication factory: a prospective study. *Contact Dermatitis* 1994; **31**:111–115.

3. Alomar A, Occupational skin disease from cutting fluids. *Dermatol Clin* 1994; **12**:537–546.

4. Mager Stellmann J, *Encyclopaedia of occupational health and safety*, 3rd revised edn. Geneva: International Labour Office; 1983.

5. Crow KD, The engineering and chemical aspects of soluble oils. *Br J Dermatol* 1981; **105(suppl. 21)**:11–18.

6. Grattan CEH, English JSC, Foulds IS, Rycroft RJG, Cutting fluid dermatitis. *Contact Dermatitis* 1989; **20**:372–376.

7. De Boer EM, van Ketel WG, Bruynzeel DP, Dermatoses in metal workers (I). Irritant contact dermatitis. *Contact Dermatitis* 1989; **20**:212–218.

8. De Boer EM, Bruynzeel DP, Occupational dermatitis by metalworking fluids. In: Menné T, Maibach HI, eds. *Hand eczema*. Boca Raton: CRC Press; 1994:217–230.

9. Zugerman C, Cutting fluids. Their use and effects on the skin. In: Adams RA, ed. *Occupational skin disease. Occupational medicine: State of the art reviews*, vol. 1, no. 2. Philadelphia: Hanley and Belfus Inc; 1986:245–258.

10. Coenraads P-J, Diepgen TL, Risk for hand eczema in employees with past or present atopic dermatitis. *Int Arch Occup Environ Health* 1998; **71**:7–13.

11. Meding B, Swanbeck G, Predictive factors for hand eczema. *Contact Dermatitis* 1990; **23**:154–161.

12. Nilsson EJ, Knutsson A, Atopic dermatitis, nickel sensitivity and xerosis as risk factors for hand eczema in women. *Contact Dermatitis* 1995; **33**:401–406.

13. Hermal, *Die Diagnostik der Kontaktallergie. Basiswissen und spezielle Informationen zu Kontaktallergenen*, 3rd revised edn. Reinbek: Hermal; 1997.

14. Geier J, Kleinhans D, Peters KP, Contact allergy due to industrial biocides. Results of the IVDK and the German Contact Dermatitis Research Group. *Dermatosen Occup Environ* 1996; **44**:154–159.

Food-processing Industry

Andrea Bauer

Intolerance reactions to food, food additives and other contacts occurring in the workplace are common job-related diseases in the food processing industry. Allergic bronchial asthma of bakers due to flour dust is probably the major health problem in this trade; skin problems definitely rank second if not first. Among them irritation is more common than allergic sensitization. The discussion given below will focus on a few special fields in this occupational division.

Table 10.5 lists some of the common irritants in the food processing industry.

Table 10.5 Irritants in the food-processing industry

Acetic acid	Fruit juice
Ascorbinic acid	Lactic acid
Bleaching reagents	Potassium bicarbonate
Calcium acetate and sulphate	Potassium iodide and bromate
Emulsifying agents	Wet dough
Enzymes	Yeast

Bakers, confectioners and related professions

Statistical reports of occupational diseases show a high incidence for work-related diseases in bakers and confectioners (Figure 10.3). In 1996, the social insurance institution for the food industry and related professions in Germany (Berufsgenossenschaft für Nahrungsmittel und Gaststätten) registered 1165 cases of occupational hand dermatitis. Bakers, confectioners and related professions accounted for 41.5%. Comparing the risk of developing occupational skin disease, bakers had the highest risk, followed by cooks and confectioners.[1]

Initially most of the affected employees show irritant contact dermatitis (ICD) on hands and forearms, because of wet work and contact to irritants such as cleaners and disinfectants, as well as the multiple skin cleansing procedures during work. The irritant effects of dough and fruits, or heat exposure from the oven are less important for the development of hand dermatitis. A prospective epidemiological cohort study in 79 baker apprentices revealed mild-to-moderate irritant hand dermatitis in 29.1% (n = 23) of the apprentices after 6 months of training.[2] Consecutive development of contact allergy or protein contact dermati-

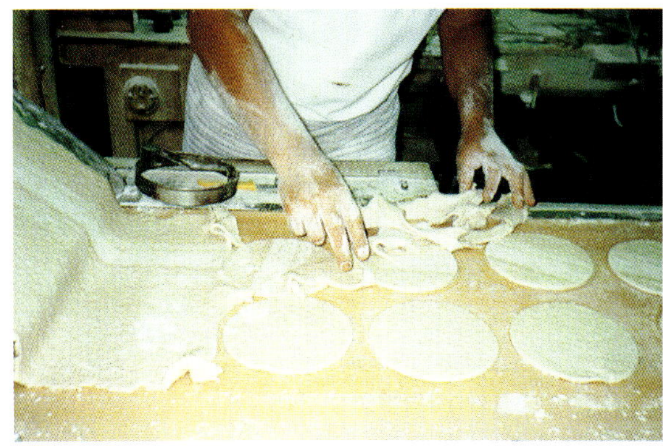

Figure 10.3: Baker's workplace.

tis after some years of working are rare in general but important to the individual. In an analysis of the 4 years patch test data from bakers recorded in the information network of dermatological clinics in Germany (IVDK), ICD due to occupational contactants was found to be more frequent than allergic contact dermatitis (ACD).[3] Type IV sensitization may lead to protein contact dermatitis and ACD. Immediate urticarial reactions and protein contact dermatitis are caused by the same proteinaceous allergens. Among them are flour, baking enzymes, fruits, milk and egg proteins, as well as mites. ACD may be caused by flavouring agents, spices, lemon peel, flour additives, antioxidants and food colourings.[4] The role of fragrances and spices in bakers' allergic contact dermatitis was investigated 20 years ago.[5] Sensitization to fragrances can be revealed by testing the fragrance mix from a standard test tray and its constituents. Regarding the high frequency of fragrance sensitization, it is hard to prove the relevance of this allergy for occupational diseases because of non-occupational exposure.

The first line candidates for ACD to spices are anise, cinnamon, vanilla, nutmeg, ginger, clove and cardamom.[6,7] Gallates (dodecylgallate, octylgallate, etc.) are used as antioxidants in fat-containing products. In some cases they have been proved to be relevant contact allergens.[8,9] The same is true for butylhydroxyanisole and butylhydroxytoluole. Persulphates and benzoyl peroxide have only historical relevance;[10] in the early 1930s they were forbidden in Denmark and The Netherlands, with a consecutive decrease in the rate of sensitization among bakers.[11] Twenty years later Germany and most other European countries also prohibited persulphates and benzoyl peroxide in the food industry. Nowadays these allergens are irrelevant for bakers and confectioners.

The evaluation of contact allergies has shown that there is no clear pattern of contactants for bakers and food handlers.[3] Thus there is no recommended specific screening tray for these professions as this would not increase the likelihood of detecting a contact allergy in the individual. Nevertheless, occupation-adapted standard patch testing is necessary. The test allergens recommended by

Table 10.6 Baker's tray

Substance	*Concentration (% pet)*
Ammoniumpersulphate	2.5
Oil of aniseed	10
Benzoylperoxide	1
Ammonium carbonate	5
Potassium bromate	5
Menthol	1
Vanilla	5

the German Contact Dermatitis Research Group (DKG) for bakers and confectioners is are given in Table 10.6.

In the differential diagnosis of contact allergy in bakers and confectioners one has to consider *Candida* and bacterial infection with consecutive development of dermatitis, paronychia and nail destruction (Figure 10.4).

Cheese makers

Very few data have been published on occupational dermatoses in cheese makers. Cheese making involves a lot of manual work. In cheese makers, sodium chloride

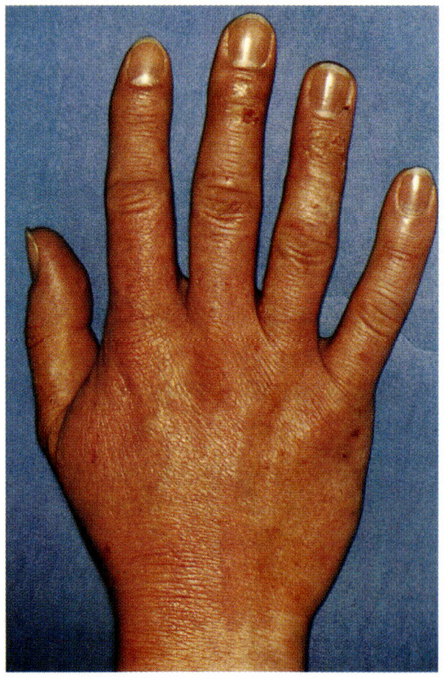

Figure 10.4: Protein CD in a baker.

up to 20% and milk proteins are the important irritants that come into direct contact with the skin. Another important factor is the wet workload of these employees, resulting in ICD. ACD, as well as protein contact dermtitis, is rare but has to be considered.[12]

References

1. Tacke J, Schmidt A, Fartasch M, Diepgen TL, Occupational contact dermatitis in bakers, confectioners and cooks. *Contact Dermatitis* 1995; **33**:112–117.
2. Bauer A, Bartsch R, Stadeler M et al., Development of occupational skin diseases during vocational training in baker and confectioner apprentices – a follow-up study. *Contact Dermatitis*, 1998; **39**:307–11.
3. Gebhardt M, Wollina U, Stadeler M, Schneider W, Zur Bedeutung der Kontaktekzeme im Bäckerhandwerk. *Arbeitsmed Sozialmed Umweltmed* 1997; **32**:431–434.
4. Rycroft RJG, Menne T, Frosch PJ, eds., *Textbook of contact dermatitis*, 2nd edn. Berlin: Springer; 1995:378.
5. Malten KE, Four bakers showing positive patch tests to a number of fragrance materials, which can also be used as flavours. *Acta Derm Venereol* 1979; **suppl 85**:117.
6. Adams RM, ed., *Occupational skin disease*, 2nd edn. Philadelphia: WB Saunders; 1990:587–588.
7. Frosch PJ, Pilz B, Peiler D et al., Die Epikutantestung mit patienteneigenen Produkten. In: Plewig G, Przybilla B, eds. *Fortschritte der praktischen Dermatologie und Venerologie.* Berlin: Springer; 1996:166–181.
8. Brun R, Eczema de contact a un antioxydant de la margarine (gallate) et changement de metier. *Dermatologica* 1970; **140**:390–394.
9. Hausen BM, Beyer W, The sensitizing capacity of the antioxidants propyl, octyl and dodecyl gallate and some related gallic acid esters. *Contact Dermatitis* 1992; **26**:253–258.
10. Wüthrich B, Zur Genese des Bäckerekzems. *Hautarzt* 1970; **21**:214–218.
11. Hjorth N, Menne T, Prevention of allergic contact sensitization: a historical perspective. In: Menne T, Maibach HI, eds. *Exogeneous dermatoses: environmental dermatitis.* Boca Raton: CRC Press; 1991:361–364.
12. Nestle FO, Elsner P, Occupational dermatoses in cheese makers: frequent association of irritant, allergic and protein contact dermatitis. *Dermatology* 1997; **194**:243–246.

HAIRDRESSERS

Andrea Bauer

Early-onset irritant contact dermatitis (ICD) in hairdressers is, to some extent, accepted to be normal by most of the employees in this profession. Erythema and scaling mostly show up on the dorsal surface of the metacarpophalangeal joint and in the web spaces between the fingers.

People with a proven atopic skin diathesis (>10 points on Diepgen's atopy score,[1] and/or a history for previous or current hand dermatitis do have a higher risk of developing hand dermatitis than do non-atopic individuals, as shown in many previous studies.[2,3] Allergic rhinitis or metal sensitization have not been shown to be significant risk factors.[2] While as a result of a recent large study of 2352 hairdressing apprentices the role of skin atopy became more controversial, unprotected wet work or dealing with irritant substances, such as shampooing, bleaching and permanent waving, remained the main significant risk factor.[4]

Occupational hand dermatitis appears early in a hair stylist's career. A cohort investigation in 224 apprentices revealed early onset hand dermatitis in 17.8% (n = 30) of the apprentices in the first 6 months of work. In view of this, prevention programmes must start early in training to prevent the onset of ICD as well as the subsequent development of allergic contact dermatitis (ACD), which is more common after some years of work. Establishing an exact allergy diagnosis is important to avoid incapacitating hand dermatitis and discontinuation of work.[2,5]

The occupational relevance of nickel sensitization for hairdressers has long been over-emphasized. Nickel data should be viewed carefully, considering concomitant factors such as the individuals' history and the manifestation of the dermatitis. In most stylists' shops, scissors and related working equipment are in any case made from stainless steel, which is not a significant source of free nickel ions.[6]

Hairdressers are exposed throughout the day to many substances with irritant and allergic properties. Shampooing, permanent waving, bleaching and dying are the main potential hazards. Glycerol monothioglycolate (GMTG) in acid permanent waves (acid perms), was found to be the most frequent occupational allergen in hairdressers: 34% were sensitized. Avoidance is difficult. This chemical penetrates latex and PVC gloves in a few seconds; only neoprene gloves are protective. Recently, some countries have tried to remove this common substance from the market. In 1997 in Germany, it was recommended in technical guidelines for hazardous materials that GMTG be replaced in permanent waves. This has already been promised by most of the big companies. As an alternative, ammoniated thiolactate has been introduced; there are no extensive data about the allergic relevance of this chemical so far. Ammonium thioglycolate in alkaline permanent waves is less allergenic; the sensitization rate was only 4% in one hairdressing unit examined.

The chemicals mentioned are essential for permanent waving to cleave the disulphide bonds of the triple helices of hair, making the hair plastic so that its configuration can be changed easily. Using ammonium persulphate for oxidizing the cysteines back to disulphide linkages renders the change permanent.[7] In higher concentrations ammonium persulphate is also used as a bleaching agent. Sensitization rates in hairdressers are up to 15.9%.[6] Besides type IV reactions, Zelger and Huber have reported immediate-type reactions in hairdressers like rhinitis, conjunctivitis, bronchial obstruction and contact urticaria after contact with persulphate.[8]

Para-phenylene diamine (PPD) which was abolished in Europe in the 1950s but is still commonly used in the USA is a marker allergen for *para* group sensitization. *Para* group substances such as *p*-toluylene diamine (PTD) are major allergens still present in hair dyes. Sensitization rates in hairdressers have been found to be 19 and 14.3%, respectively.[6]

Henna, a natural vegetable dye, has a low allergic power. The incidence of delayed-type and immediate-type hypersensitivity appears to be extremely rare. Only a few cases are reported in literature.[9] Another low-power allergen is hydrochinone, an antioxidant in hair dyes and permanent waves.

Further relevant allergens are fragrances, cocamidopropylbetaine, pyrogallole and preservatives in shampoos and hair cosmetics. In regard to cocamidopropylbetaine, irritant reactions are predominant; relevant allergic reactions are seen rarely.[10]

Current allergens in perms are ammonium thiolactate and cysteamine. As for ammonium thiolactate, no relevant data are available about the allergenic properties of cysteamine.

Protective gloves can themselves cause ACD. The main allergens are thiurame, carbamate, thiourea and benzothiazole, as dealt with on p.84. Contact urticaria and protein contact dermatitis from latex proteins are further problems caused by intolerance to protective gloves.[11]

The prognosis of occupational contact dermatitis depends on the hairdresser's personal history of previous hand dermatitis and the extent of wet work they do during the day.

Patch testing hairdressers

In the routine office patch test, a standard tray together with a hairdressers' tray may be a good first screening to use (see Table 10.7). For scientific evaluation in allergy centres or for medicolegal reasons, the patient's own products should be included in the patch tests. How to test commercial products of the individ-

Table 10.7 Patch test tray recommendation for hairdressers

Allergen	*Concentration (% pet)*	*Source*
Ammonium thioglycolate	1	Alkaline permanent wave
Ammonium persulphate	2.5	Bleaching agent
p-Toluylen diamine (freie Base)	1	Hair dye
3-Aminophenole	1	Hair dye
p-Aminophenole	1	Hair dye
Hydrochinone	1	Permanent waves/hair dye
Pyrogallol*	1	Coupling agent in dye
Glyceryl monothioglycolate†	1	Acid permanent wave
Cocamidopropylbetaine	1 (aq)	Shampoo

*Removed from market in Germany in 1993.
†Recommended for substitution in Germany in 1997.

ual patient? I recommend testing rinse-off products such as shampoos or surfactants diluted to 1% and 0.1% in water. "Leave-on" products should be tested as they are. It takes much experience to differentiate between irritant and weak positive reactions in the test reaction to a shampoo. Dilution of 1% or below risk losing a true allergic reaction because the allergen is too highly diluted. Conversely, higher concentrations are almost always irritant to the skin. In this conflict, the repeated open application test (ROAT) might be a good compromise. An exclusion test, a "use" test or workplace exposure may answer any remaining questions. Immediate-type reactions can be identified by the standard procedures (prick, scratch or intradermal test, if appropriate) followed by exposing the patient in the workplace.

References

1. Diepgen TL, Fartasch M, Hornstein OP, Kriterien zur Beurteilung des der atopischen Hautdiathese. *Derm Beruf Umwelt* 1991; **39**:79–83.

2. Bauer A, Seidel A, Bartsch R et al., Entwicklung von Hautproblemen bei Berufsanfängern in Hautrisikoberufen. *Allergologie* 1997; **20**:179–183.

3. Uter W, Gefeller O, Schwanitz HJ, Einfluß von Hautempfindlichkeit und Arbeitsschutzmaßnahmen auf die Manifestation von Berufsekzemen bei Friseuren. Erste Ergebnisse einer prospektiven Kohortenstudie. *Allergologie* 1994; **18**:312–315.

4. Uter W, Pfahlberg A, Gefeller O, Schwanitz HJ, Risk factors for hand dermatitis in hairdressers apprentices. *Dermatosen* 1998; **46**:151–158.

5. Majoie IML, Von Blomberg BME, Bruynzeel DP, Development of hand eczema in junior hairdressers: an 8-year follow-up study. *Contact Dermatitis* 1996; **34**:243–247.

6. Frosch PJ, Burrows D, Camarasa JG et al., Reactions to a hairdressers'series: results from 9 European centres. The European environmental and contact dermatitis research group (EECDRG). *Contact Dermatitis* 1993; **28**:180–183.

7. Storrs FJ, Permanent wave contact dermatitis: contact allergy to glyceryl monothioglycolate. *J Am Acad Dermatol* 1984; **11**:74–85.

8. Zelger J, Huber W, Inhalationsallergie durch Meche-Breie im Friseurgewerbe. *Derma Beruf Umwelt* 1989; **37**:220–221.

9. Garcia Ortiz JC, Terron M, Bellido J, Contact allergy to henna. *Int Arch Allergy Immunol* 1997; **114**:298–299.

10. De Groot AC, Van der Walle HB, Weyland JW, Contact allergy to cocamidopropyl betaine. *Contact Dermatitis* 1995; **33**:419–422.

11. Van der Walle HB, Brunsveld VM, Latex allergy among hairdressers. *Contact Dermatitis* 1995; **32**:117.

CONSTRUCTION WORKERS

Matthias Gebhardt

Classically, construction workers were bricklayers who were exposed to cement and irritants such as dust and dirt. Nowadays, with increasing requirements for mechanical properties of the buildings, easiness of handling and introduction of modern synthetic materials this profession has changed quite a lot. Moreover, because of long-standing economic crises, many construction workers are unemployed from time to time and change their job profiles and hence their exposure situation continuously. Therefore, it may be rather difficult to follow up previous exposure situations in an occupational case history. Nevertheless, classical allergens such as chromate in cement have not lost their importance yet.

Cement

Cement is a powder mainly consisting of calcium oxide (lime), which is transformed to calcium hydroxide (slaked lime) by adding water. Concrete or mortar contain approximately 10–20% cement. In moist conditions, cement it is a strong alkaline substance with a pH reaching 12. Contact with wet cement can therefore cause cement burns, which may develop hours after exposure and may result in necrosis of the skin. In dermatological terms this is an acute toxic contact dermatitis. The overlying skin of the knees and the feet (if cement enters the boots) are commonly affected.

In addition to its alkaline character, cement can irritate the skin by its hygroscopic properties. It dries up the skin, making it cracked, fissured and, as a consequence, thickened. Such a cement eczema has been well known for centuries. Constant damage to the epidermal barrier paves the way for subsequent development of allergy. Allergic contact dermatitis (ACD) usually appears after years of work with cement. Chromium salts are the allergenic compounds in cement. To elicit contact dermatitis, cement powder has to be moistened; contact with moistened cement may result from touching the wet cement during the work process or from sweat-induced dampening of skin – contaminating the cement powder. Cement dust sticks to the fabric of the clothing worn by construction workers and therefore can cause widespread distribution of dermatitis. Finished concrete constructions are non-sensitizing.

Positive patch test reactions to chromate were first reported in 1939 by Bonnevie. Hexavalent chromium salts in cement are much stronger sensitizers than Cr(III) salts. Chromate dermatitis is the main occupational skin disease in

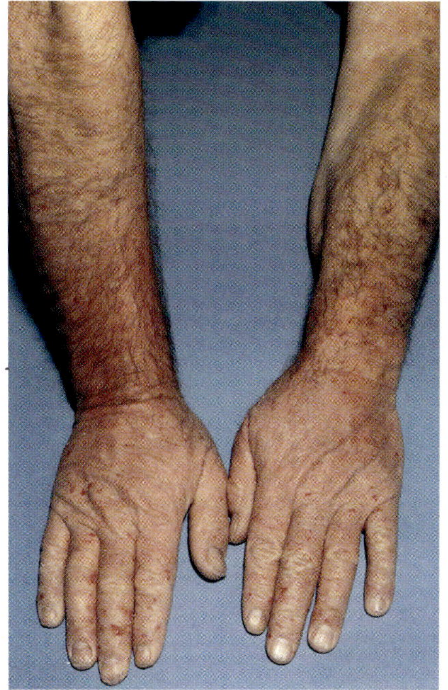

Figure 10.5: Chronic ACD reaction to chromate in cement.

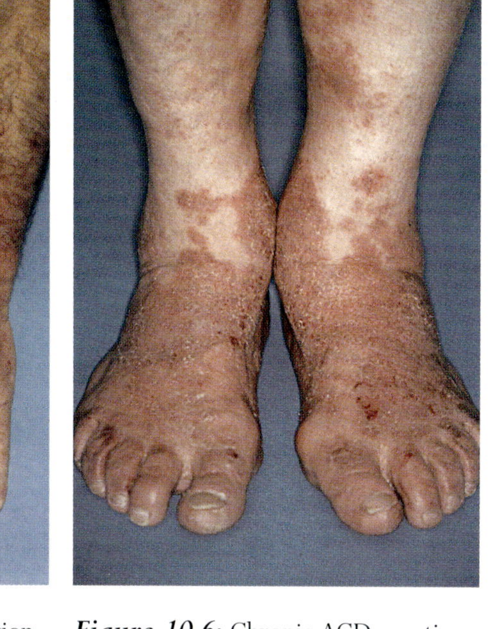

Figure 10.6: Chronic ACD reaction to chromate in cement.

bricklayers, workers in the manufacture of pre-fabricated concrete parts and related trades (Figures 10.5 and 10.6). Today, with an increasing number of people undertaking home building projects, cement eczema is increasingly explained by the leisure-time activities of hobbiest construction workers. In a recent German study, chromate was the main occupational allergen in construction workers accounting for 44% patch test positivity of male construction workers compared with 4% in the male population without a construction background.[1]

Hexavalent chromium is formed from trivalent raw material chromium during the heating process in modern kilns. By adding ferrous sulphate to cement, the allergenicity of chromate can be lowered by transforming Cr(VI) back into Cr(III) salts.[2] This is a very important finding, which has been successfully exploited, starting in Scandinavian countries, especially Denmark, in the 1980s.[3] The number of chromate allergies decreased significantly with this preventive measure.[4] However, there are some remaining single cases who still develop ACD and this measure has no effect on irritant properties of cement.[4,5]

Chromate sensitization may develop after years of cement contact and typically becomes chronic.[6] The prognosis of chromate dermatitis is bad. It seems to persist for years even without further contact. The consecutive development of cutaneous T-cell lymphoma in chromate allergics has been controversially discussed by some authors. Cutaneous T-cell lymphoma in construction workers should be discussed in the context of possible persistent allergenic boost maintained by chromate, but final conclusions have not been made yet.[7] However, if strict avoidance of chromate can be guaranteed by job change or retirement, a fairly good outcome is possible. In a study of Swiss construction workers sensitized to chromate and with a declaration of medical inability, 72% were free of skin lesions within the first 5 years of enforcement of avoidance measures.[8]

Rubber chemicals

Among relevant occupational allergens of construction workers rubber chemicals play a controversial role. Rubber gloves and boots are worn to avoid skin contact with hazardous substances such as wet cement, however they are allergenic themselves. Construction workers are significantly more numerous among those individuals reacting to rubber chemicals than are members of other occupations. Thiurams and carbamates are the typical allergens in this group.[9] An unexpected exposure may be the use of thiurams as preservatives in tile-fixing adhesives.

Plastics

Whereas cement was the most important cause of irritant and allergic disorders formerly, nowadays plastics are gaining importance. Synthetic materials are added to building materials in order to improve properties such as stability, corrosion resistance and ease of procession. Epoxy resins are of special interest for these purposes. They are used as adhesives for fixing tiles and, therefore, epoxy resins may be an occupational allergen for tilers. In an investigation of epoxy resin allergy among exposed construction workers, one-fifth were found to be positive to epoxy resin or resin hardeners.[10] Only half of them had experienced skin problems before.

Another common exposure is floor coverings in heavily frequented areas such as public buildings, hospitals, laboratory rooms, supermarkets, etc. Only a few construction workers are employed in companies that specialize in such flooring work. These workers are highly exposed to epoxy resins and, if sensitized, may be heavily affected with severe contact dermatitis that requires sick leave.[11] Consequently, strict skin protection against epoxy resin contact is required; it is worth noting that gloves made of fabric or cotton are dangerous because they soak up the liquid allergenic materials and artificially prolong the skin exposure.

When patch tested, epoxy workers are likely to react to different epoxy resins, bis-acrylates and hardeners. Among the hardeners various amines are of allergic importance and are available from most patch test providers. Diaminodiphenyl methane, hexamethylene diamine and isophorone diamine have been found superior among construction workers compared to the normal population, which indicates the relevance of those hardeners.[1] Insulation foams based on polyurethane are used by many construction trades. Isocyanate components used in processing these foams are allergically relevant, most of all as IgE-mediated allergens for the respiratory tract in isocyanate asthma.

Other

ICD can also be elicited by working with mineral fibre such as mineral insulation wool. The time of exposure correlated well with symptoms in the skin, eyes and upper respiratory tract in a Danish study.[12] Patch tests with mineral wool are pointless; the irritant nature of the complaints is obvious. Concrete casting oils and stone cleansers, mostly acids, have been reported by others as possible irritants (Figure 10.7).[13]

An interesting observation has been made by Skogstad and Levy, who reported fungal infections to *Trichophyton rubrum* on the hands of four construction workers.[14] Although the fungal infection in these cases was accompanied by tinea pedis, there may also have been an association with ICD. The impaired epidermal barrier may facilitate the invasion of infectious agents such as dermatophytes).

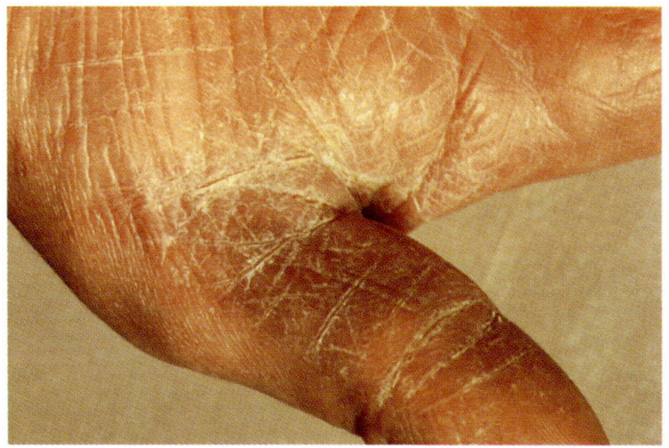

Figure 10.7: ICD of the hand (detail).

Conclusion

The test trays recommended in Table 10.8 should be considered when patch testing construction workers. Many relevant allergens are already included in the standard series. Plastics should always be included in the screening. Preservatives are not only important in industrial coolants but also in barrier creams and skin cleansers used among the workers. One can easily overlook special and rare sensitization such as textile dyes from working suits, airborne plant allergens and woods. These should be tested and ruled out when no other relevant allergen is found. Atopic dermatitis will commonly flare, reappear or first manifest in construction workers due to irritant exposure.

Table 10.8 Test spectrum for construction workers; samples from the workplace should only be used with great caution (danger of active sensitization)

Standard tray	Potassium dichromate Epoxy resin Rubber chemicals Paraphenylenediamine (IPPD)
Plastics	Hardeners Formaldehyde resins Isocyanates Methacrylates
Preservatives	Skin protection creams Skin cleansers

References

1. Geier J, Schnuch A, Kontaktallergien im Bauhauptgewerbe. *Dermatosen* 1998; **36**:109–114.

2. Avnstorp C, Cement eczema. In: Menne T, Maibach HI, eds. *Exogenous dermatoses: environmental dermatitis*. Boca Raton: CRC Press; 1991:401–414.

3. Avnstorp C, Cement eczema: an epidemiological intervention study. *Acta Derm Venereol (Stockh)* 1992; **suppl 179**:1–22.

4. Bruze M, Gruvberger B, Hradil E, Chromate sensitization and elicitation from cement with iron sulfate. *Acta Derm Venereol* 1990; **70**:160–162.

5. Avnstorp C, Prevalence of cement eczema in Denmark before and since addition of ferrous sulfate to Danish cement. *Acta Derm Venereol* 1989; **69**:151–155.

6. Hogan DJ, Dannaker CJ, Maibach HI, The prognosis of contact dermatitis. *J Am Acad Dermatol* 1990; **23**:300–307.

7. Fisher AA, Testifying in medicolegal cases involving dermatoses of possible exogenous origin. In: Menne T, Maibach HI, eds. *Exogenous dermatoses: environmental dermatitis.* Boca Raton: CRC Press; 1991:262–266.

8. Lips R, Rast H, Elsner P, Outcome of job change in patients with occupational chromate dermatitis. *Contact Dermatitis* 1996; **34**:268–271.

9. Conde-Salazar L, del Rio E, Guimaraens D, Gonzalez de Domingo MA, Type IV allergy to rubber additives: a 10 year study of 686 cases. *J Am Acad Dermatol* 1993; **29**:176–180.

10. van Putten PB, Coenraads PJ, Nater JP, Hand dermatoses and contact allergic reactions in construction workers exposed to epoxy resins. *Contact Dermatitis* 1984; **10**:146–150.

11. Conde-Salazar L, Gonzalez de Domingo MA, Guimaraens D, Sensitization to epoxy resin systems in special flooring workers. *Contact Dermatitis* 1994; **31**:157–160.

12. Petersen R, Sabroe S, Irritative symptoms and exposure to mineral wool. *Am J Ind* 1991; **20**:113–122.

13. Geier J, Struppek K, Anamnese-Auxilium für die berufsdermatologische Untersuchung von Maurern, Betonbauern, Fliesenlegern und Angehörigen verwandter Berufe. *Dermatosen* 1995; **43**:75–80.

14. Skogstad M, Levy F, Occupational irritant contact dermatitis and fungal infection in construction workers. *Contact Dermatitis* 1994; **31**:28–30.

11. DISINFECTANTS, ANTISEPTICS AND ANTIMICROBIALS

Undine Berndt and Peter Elsner

Infectious skin diseases are a very common clinical problem resulting in an extensive use of topical antibiotics and antiseptics. As the application of these substances may be accompanied by side-effects that may greatly endanger the patient, topical antimicrobial preparations should be used only when there are strong indications. Side-effects can induce contact sensitization, local and, due to resorption, systemic toxic effects, and the development of antibiotic-resistant strains of micro-organisms.

Topical antibiotics

Topical antibiotics are among the most frequently prescribed medications in dermatology. They also are one of the most common causes of allergic contact dermatitis (ACD). Thirty per cent of all patients with leg ulcers[1,2] and 15% of patients suffering from external otitis[3] are sensitized, presumably secondary to long-term exposure to frequent applications of antibiotic to an altered cutaneous barrier.[4] Antibiotics are usually present in a number of commercially available ointments and creams that are used on minor cuts and abrasions as well as post-surgical wounds.

Neomycin is the oldest but still frequently used topical antibiotic of the aminoglycoside group. It belongs to the most frequently encountered topical sensitizers. The prevalence of neomycin sensitization in the general population is close to 1%.[4,5] Patients suffering from stasis dermatitis and leg ulcers are commonly sensitive to neomycin (20–30%). In a study of patients who had post-surgical wound treatment, approximately 5% showed a positive patch-test result when exposed to neomycin.[6] Besides the more common delayed-type hypersensitivity reactions, neomycin induces mast-cell degranulation, resulting in anaphylactic reactions.[7,8] Crossreactivity to other aminoglycosides such as gentamicin has been observed. This carries the danger of allergic reactions if a systemic administration of gentamicin is necessary in the case of a life-threatening situation, such as septicaemia.

Another example for an antibiotic with a strong potential for sensitization is bacitracin, a polypeptide antibiotic. As well as type IV contact dermatitis, urticaria and anaphylaxis have been described.[9,10]

Sulphonamides are very potent sensitizers too.[11] After topical treatment they may cause contact dermatitis, erythema multiforme or photosensitization to UV

B. Up to 9% of people using topical sulphonamides develop allergic reactions. A further problem is crossreactivity to chemically related diuretic and antidiabetic substances.

Antibiotics with relatively rare side-effects when used topically are erythromycin, tetracycline, sodium fusidate and polymyxin.[12]

Antiseptics and disinfectants

Antiseptics are used on the skin to prevent the spread of micro-organisms and to prevent post-operative infection. They reduce the count of micro-organisms in skin diseases that are known to be complicated by a high microbial load, such as atopic dermatitis. Concentrations must be low in order to prevent irritant contact dermatitis and toxic side-effects due to transcutaneous resorption. The same substances, although in higher concentrations and thus with microbicidal effect, are used as disinfectants. The most commonly used substances belong to the groups of halogen compounds, heavy metal compounds, oxidants and dyes.[13] Besides their local irritation potential, they may also be contact sensitizers. Clioquinol,[14,15] thiomersal,[16] and benzoyl peroxide[17] are frequently encountered examples. Dyes, such as ethacridin may cause photosensitization.

While dermatitis due to the application of antiseptics is mostly seen in surgical or dermatologic patients; disinfectants are a well-known cause of occupational contact dermatitis in health care and hospital cleaning personnel. The most common type of contact dermatitis in these occupations is of irritant character due to the high frequency of contact with water, detergents and disinfectant solutions. This irritation may provoke allergic sensitization to one or more of the considerable number of substances with sensitizing potential, such as formaldehyde or glutaraldehyde and chloramine.[18–20]

Biocides and preservatives

Topical preparations and household, industrial and other products must be protected against the deterioration that can be caused by micro-organisms. This problem is solved by the addition of antimicrobials to a product, such as alcohols, mercurial compounds, parabens, phenolic compounds, quarternary ammonium compounds, quinoline derivatives, tocopherol and triphenylmethane dyes.[13] These substances may cause contact dermatitis, especially when used on already damaged skin. They are often identified as causative agents in occupational contact dermatitis, e.g. due to metal-working fluids. However, taking into account their widespread presence, the overall impact of most preservatives on public health must be considered low.

References

1. Wilson CI, Cameron J, Powell SM et al., High incidence of contact dermatitis in leg-ulcer patients – implications for management. *Clin Exp Dermatol* 1991; **16**: 250–253.

2. Zaki I, Shall L, Dalziel KL, Bacitracin: a significant sensitizer in leg ulcer patients? *Contact Dermatitis* 1994; **31**:92–94.

3. Van Ginkel CJW, Bruintjes TD, Huizing EH, Allergy due to topical medications in chronic otitis externa and chronic otitis media. *Clin Otolaryngol* 1995; **20**: 326–328.

4. Rietschel RL, Dermatologic manifestations of antimicrobial adverse reactions with special emphasis on topical exposure. *Infect Dis N Am* 1994; **8**: 607–615.

5. Prystowsky SD, Nonomura Jh, Smith RW, Allen AM, Allergic hypersensitivity to neomycin. Relationship between patch test reactions and use tests. *Arch Dermatol* 1979; **115**:713–715.

6. Gette MT, Marks JG, Maloney ME, Frequency of postoperative allergic contact dermatitis to topical antibiotics. *Arch Dermatol* 1992; **128**:365–367.

7. Simon C, Stille W, Lokalantibiotika. In: Simon S, Stille W, eds. *Antibiotika-Therapie in Klinik und Praxis*, 8th edn. Stuttgart: Schattauer; 1993: 207–213.

8. Proebstle TM, Jugert FK, Merk HF, Gall H, Severe anaphylactic reaction to topical administration of framycetin. *J Allergy Clin Immunol* 1995; **96**:429–430.

9. Held JL, Kalb RE, Ruszkowski AM, DeLeo V, Allergic contact dermatitis from bacitracin. *J Am Acad Dermatol* 1987; **17**:592–594.

10. Elsner P, Pevny I, Burg G, Anaphylaxis induced by topically applied bacitracin. *Am J Contact Dermatitis* 1990; **1**:162–164.

11. McKenna SR, Latenser BA, Jones LM et al., Serious silver sulfadiazine and mafedine acetate dermatitis. *Burns* 1995; **21**:310–312.

12. Nater JP, DeGroot AC, *Unwanted effects of cosmetics and drugs used in dermatology*, 2nd edn. Amsterdam: Elsevier; 1985:67–72.

13. Höger PH, Topische Antibiotica und Antiseptika. *Hautarzt* 1998; **49**:331–347.

14. Goh CL, Contact sensitivity to topical antimicrobials (I). Epidemiology in Singapore. *Contact Dermatitis* 1989; **21**:46–48.

15. Wantke F, Gotz M, Jarisch R, Contact dermatitis from cloxyquin. *Contact Dermatitis* 1995; **32**:112–113.

16. Ancona A, Arevalo A, Macotela E, Contact dermatitis in hospital patients. *Dermatol Clin* 1990; **8**:95–105.

17. Chren MM, Bickers DR, Dermatological pharmacology. In: Goodman Gilman A, Rall TW, Nies AS, Taylor P, eds. *The pharmacological basis of therapeutics*. New York: Pergamon Press; 1990:1572–1591.

18. Goossens A, Claes L, Drieghe J, Put E, Antimicrobials, preservatives, antiseptics and disinfectants. *Contact Dermatitis* 1997; **39**:133–134.

19. Hansen KS, Occupational dermatoses in hospital cleaning women. *Contact Dermatitis* 1983; **9**:343–351.

20. Rudzki E, Rebandel P, Grzywa Z, Patch tests with occupational contactants in nurses, doctors and dentists. *Contact Dermatitis* 1989; **20**:247–50.

12. Cosmetic Intolerance

Undine Berndt and Peter Elsner

Generally, cosmetic products are applied to the skin for long time periods, and often to large skin areas of the body. Cosmetic products are applied to the skin for long time periods and often to large skin areas of the body. The product is used as a leave-on or a rinse-off cosmetic even in very delicate parts of the body such as the moist and warm environment of body folds. In all of these circumstances a cosmetic product should not cause irritant or allergic reactions on the skin when used for the designated purpose. Consequently, the European Commission demands safety tests for all cosmetics before their introduction to the market.[1] Despite their widespread use, serious adverse effects caused by cosmetics and toiletry products are infrequent. For each one million items sold, 10–200 cases of irritation, allergy, photosensitization or acne are seen each year.[2] Mild reactions, such as itching, prickling or dryness, however, may occur in more than 10% of the adult population.[3]

Irritation

Irritant contact dermatitis is the most commonly encountered adverse reaction to cosmetics and skin-care products. Personal cleanliness products, such as soaps, shampoo, bath foam and deodorants are the most important irritants.[4,5] Irritation may occur immediately after a single skin application, showing signs of acute contact dermatitis, such as erythema, oedema and vesicles. This type of inflammation is a rare situation and generally requires contact with rather strong irritants, which cosmetics are not. More frequently skin damage results from a chronic cumulative or repetitive irritation with only sub-threshold effects.

Irritancy is not only a matter of the irritant capacity of a given product and concentration of the irritant agent. It also depends on the duration, mode and rate of application, and it is complicated by inter-individual variability in skin resistance. People who already have impaired stratum corneum barrier function, such as atopics, elderly patients or people with compromized skin due to occupational hazards, are predisposed to irritant reactions to cosmetics.

In contrast to the clinically evaluable forms of irritation, which are characterized by objective signs of inflammation, subjective irritation may occur; this is a non-inflammatory response of some individuals to externally applied preparations. It is characterized by sensory discomfort, such as tingling, tightness, pruritus and burning without visible skin changes. These symptoms may be noticed immediately following the application or delayed by minutes, hours or days. In some cases, sensory irritation only occurs after application of product combinations. According to surveys of cosmetic manufacturer surveys, 1–10% of facial cosmetic users experience these subjective perceptions.[6] The affected persons or so-called stingers can be selected by special test methods, triggering the symptoms by the topical application of organic acids, e.g. lactic acid.[7] "Status cosmeticus" is a term created by Fisher which describes a condition in which patients try many cosmetics and complain of being unable to tolerate any of them.[8]

Allergies

Contact allergic reactions make up less than 10% of all unwanted effects from cosmetic products. The prevalence rates of positive patch-test reactions indicating a sensitization to cosmetics are approximately 4% in European countries and the USA.[3,9] The most commonly involved product categories as determined by the North American Contact Dermatitis Group and by the European dermatology community are skin care products, nail and hair cosmetics, make-ups and fragrance products. Preservatives, fragrances, emulsifiers, vehicles and colourants are frequently implicated as sensitizers.[3,4,9]

Sensitization to cosmetics is assisted if the skin is already compromized. The most frequently affected body site is the face (e.g. see Figure 12.1). Clinical manifestations range from pruritus to a classic contact dermatitis that occurs, at its earliest, 24 hours after contact and presents a polymorphous clinical picture. The localization usually gives information on the related agent, e.g. cheilitis as result of lipstick application, although skin lesions sometimes arise at distant areas of the body, such as eczema of the eyelid caused by nail-polish sensitization.

The diagnosis of cosmetic allergy is usually based on a positive patch test to a product. Besides the standard series, which includes the most familiar allergens, specific test batteries and the patient's own cosmetic products suspected

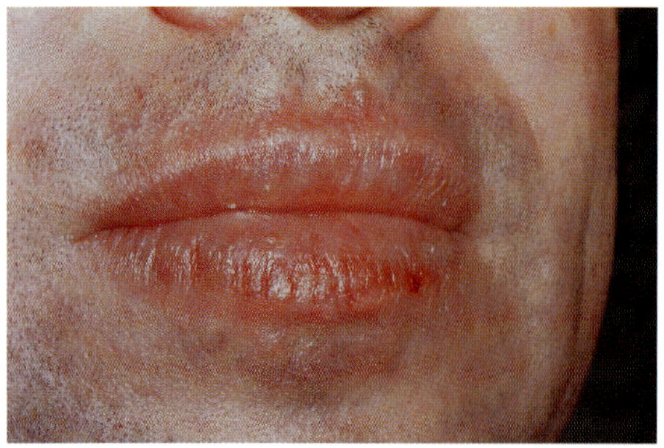

Figure 12.1: Allergic contact dermatitis due to lipstick.

to cause allergic symptoms give valuable information. Additionally, a positive "use" test or repeated open application test (ROAT) may lead to the diagnosis. Once an allergen is identified as a causative agent its use has to be avoided. Therefore it is of paramount importance that a complete qualitative declaration of all constituents of cosmetics is given by manufacturers. The patient should be informed about his or her sensitization using the International Nomenclature of Cosmetic Ingredients (INCI) terminology which is used in the USA and Europe.

Photosensitization

The third most common category of side-effects due to cosmetics are photosensitivity reactions. These may be of phototoxic or photoallergic character. Phototoxic substances, such as coumarins and furocoumarins, are present in various perfumes and exaggerate the cutaneous non-immunological response to exposure to sunlight. In contrast, photoallergic reactions require sensitization. Constituents of cosmetics can be modified by sunlight, which may result in a transformation to an antigen responsible for allergy. Photosensitization often causes hyperpigmentation. As it is mostly perfumes that are involved, this is usually localized in the neck and *décolletage* region or is retroauricular.[2]

Other dermatoses

Cosmetics may aggravate pre-existing dermatoses, such as seborrhoic dermatitis, acne or rosacea. Furthermore, cosmetics containing comedonic compounds, e.g. petrolatum in excessively greasy preparations such as night creams, may cause acneiform eruptions. The age of the patient suggests the cause, as the most affected females are beyond the acne age. The patient usually does not blame her cosmet-

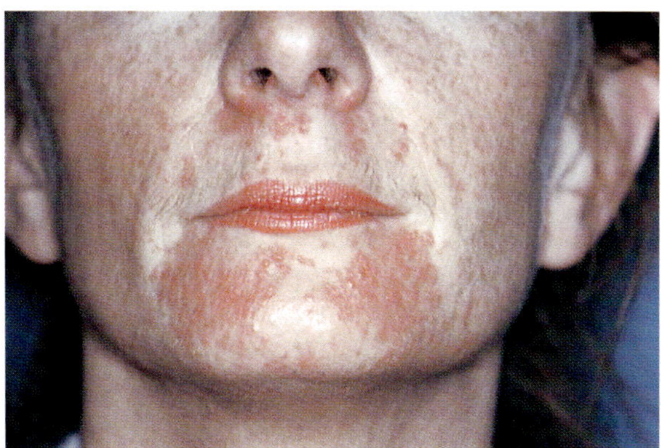

Figure 12.2: Perioral dermatitis caused by an excessive use of moisturizing creams.

ics, she often even uses them more frequenty than before, which leads to a vicious circle. Comedogenicity and acnegenicity do not depend only on the ingredients of the product but also on the susceptibility of a person to develop comedonal plugs. Cosmetics that cause acne in one person do not necessarily do so in others.[10] Perioral dermatitis, a dermatosis of not entirely clear aetiology, is often observed in patients who make excessive use of skin-care products, especially moisturizers (Figure 12.2). The so-called zero therapy, meaning the avoidance of all topically applied products, usually leads to a quick improvement of the skin condition.

On rare occasions, bacterial contamination of an insufficiently preserved preparation may accidentally cause infections, such as folliculitis.[11]

References

1. European Commission, Geänderter Vorschlag für eine Richtlinie des Rates zur sechsten Änderung der Richtlinie /6/768/EWG zur Angleichung der Rechtsvorschriften der Mitgliedsstaaten über kosmetische Mittel. *Amtsblatt Eur Gem* 1992; **C249**:5–18.
2. Meynardier J, Meynardier JM, Marck Y, True cosmetic-induced dermatitis. In: Baran R, Maibach HI, eds. *Cosmetic dermatology*. London: Martin Dunitz; 1994:551–556.
3. De Groot AC, Bruynzeel P, Bos JD, van der Meeren HLM et al., The allergens in cosmetics. *Arch Dermatol* 1988; **124**:1525–1529.
4. De Groot AC, Contact allergy to cosmetics: causative ingredients. *Contact Dermatitis* 1987;**17**:26–34.
5. Broeckx W, Blondeel A, Dooms-Goossens A, Achten G, Cosmetic intolerance. *Contact Dermatitis* 1987; **16**:189–194.
6. Amin S, Maibach HI, Cosmetic intolerance syndrome: pathophysiology and management. *Cosmetic Dermatol* 1996; **9**:34–42.
7. Draelos ZD, Sensitive skin: perceptions, evaluation, and treatment. *Am J Contact Dermatitis* 1997;**8**:67–78.
8. Fisher AA, Cosmetic actions and reactions: therapeutic, irritant and allergic. *Cutis* 1980; **26**:22–29.
9. Adams RM, Maibach HI, A five-year study of cosmetic reactions. *J Am Acad Dermatol* 1985; **13**:189–194.
10. Draelos Z, *Cosmetics in dermatology*, 2nd edn. New York: Churchill Livingstone; 1995:261–276.
11. Trüeb RM, Elsner P, Burg G, *Pseudomonas-aeruginosa*-Follikulitis nach Epilation. *Hautarzt* 1993;**44**:103–105.

13. TEXTILE DERMATITIS

Walter Wigger-Alberti

Textiles make us more independent of our environment and changes in climate. On the one hand they protect skin from the environment; on the other hand they are themselves a fashioned environment that may cause damage to the skin and body. Severe textile dermatitis is considered to be rare, in view of the vast production of clothing. Reports of dermatitis due to clothing usually describe sporadic oligosymptomatic cases or minor epidemics only. However, because complaints are mainly minor, such as diffuse itching of the affected skin only, the occurrence may be underestimated and more systematic population-based research is needed. This chapter will focus on the wide spectrum of clinical features, the main mechanisms such as irritant contact dermatitis (ICD, often observed in atopics intolerant to wool and synthetic fibres) and allergic contact dermatitis (ACD, usually caused by textile finishes and dyes), and diagnostic problems.

Clinical features

Atopics

The intolerance of atopics to wool fibres is so common that it has been enlisted as a diagnostic pattern. Even synthetic fibres may feel unpleasant, causing itch and prickle, while cotton fibres are well tolerated. The sensations are dependent on the mean diameter of the wool fibres: fabrics containing larger diameter fibres (36mm) are rougher than fabrics with smaller diameter fibres (20mm).[1] Patients with other forms of eczema and control subjects with healthy skin, however, have the same level of comfort with both cotton and polyester fibres.

Irritant contact dermatitis

ICD due to fibres, fibreglass or textile chemicals is caused by non-specific damage of the epidermis, with a significant influence by the textile's roughness and friction. As frictional properties are dependent on skin humidity, skin areas such as the intertriginous areas are especially affected. Additionally, irritant textile dermatitis is usually located where the skin surface is damaged by hard and sharp components such as labels, causing dermatitis at the neck or the waist, or buttons and tight belts causing friction and pressure against the skin. These lesions may sometimes be pigmented or purpuric.[2]

Allergic contact dermatitis

ACD due to fibres, whether they are natural (e.g. cotton, silk or wool) or synthetic (e.g. polyamide, polyester or acrylic), is very rare and more commonly due to the dyes and finishes. Sites affected in textile dermatitis usually correspond to areas where the clothes are in close contact with the skin, such as the sides and back of the neck (collar), the margins of the axillae, the borders of the axillae, the anterior and posterior folds of the axillae, the elbow flexures, the waistline, the inner thighs, the gluteal folds and the popliteal fossae (Figure 13.1); areas without contact are spared. While the hands and arms are affected by gloves, dermatitis due to stockings and socks typically shows a sharp border where the socks end. Except when gloves are worn, the hands are the most common sites of occupationally induced textile dermatitis. Pressure, sweating and friction may enhance the provocation of lesions. A wide variety of clinical patterns has been seen in confirmed cases of contact allergy to fabric finish, dyes or other components:[3–5] typical eczematous eruptions (papules or vesicles in the acute phase, and scaling and lichenified patches in the chronic phase) or even persisitent erythematous wheal-type lesions, transient urticarial lesions or an eruption resembling erythema multiforme.

Diagnosis

When textile allergy is suspected, investigation should include both clinical examination of the patient and careful study of the article incriminated. Special attention should be given to the area of the lesions and it should be kept in mind that even contamination of textiles by an external agent may cause irritant or allergic reactions. Mostly, the patients themselves suspect clothing is playing an important role in the dermatitis, though relevant sensitization is found only in

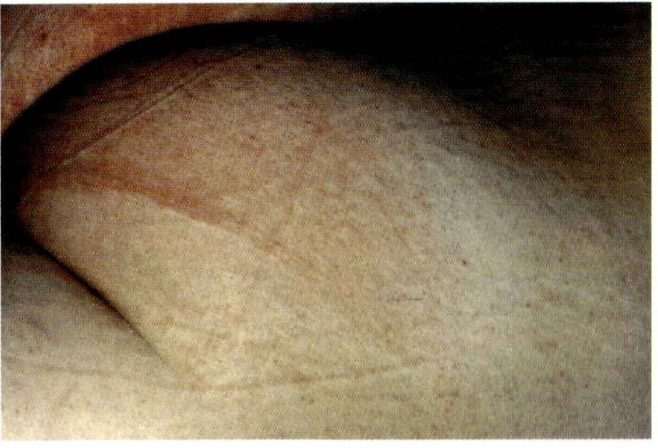

Figure 13.1: Textile dermatitis reaction to pants (no patch test).

the minority of cases. Seidenari et al.[6] noted that only 16 of 100 patients found to be sensitized to textile dyes had been suspected clinically.

In spite of very distinct intolerance to wool fibres by atopics, identification of the type of dermatitis will usually be attempted using patch tests, including a standard series. The most common textile allergens are included in commercially available extra series (e.g. Hermal, Reinbek, Germany; Chemotechnique Diagnostics AB, Malmö, Sweden). In addition to patch testing with specific textile colours and finish series, tests using some extra allergens relevant to textile, leather and fur dyes of the azo group (*p*-aminobenzene, *o*-nitro-paraphenylendiamine) have been recommended.[7]

Not only defined allergens but even the suspected textiles themselves should be tested. Therefore, pieces of fabric about 5 × 5cm are cut and fixed onto the skin, with skin contacting both the inside and the outside of the textile. Samples of the clothing materials should be soaked in water for 10–15 min before, if there is suspicion of allergy to finishes, and fixed to the skin with an overlapped sheet of tape.[5,8] In cases where dye allergy is suspected the material should be soaked for 30–60 min in acetone or ethanol.[5] If a positive reaction is found to the textile but not to the defined allergens tested, the investigator whenever possible should try to find out the actual dyes and finishes used in the textile. In practice, this is usually very difficult because only some manufacturers of textiles give information on the chemicals used; due to the great amount of imported textiles, sometimes it is impossible. Thin-layer chromatographic analysis of a specific clothing sample may be helpful to discriminate different dyes' content and after isolation, purification and epicutaneous testing the main sensitizers may be found.

If the result of testing the samples is negative, special types of patch test should be performed such as removing the stratum corneum by tape stripping before application of the patch tests or a provocation test by wearing the textile suspected ("use test"). In cases of new allergens or the patient's own samples, a panel of volunteers with healthy skin should be tested to decide between irritant and allergic reactions.

Allergens

Fibres

Fibres may cause acute or cumulative ICD or exacerbation of atopic dermatitis but cases of allergic reactions are very rare compared with allergic reactions to other causative agents. Some cases of allergy to fibre additives such as flame retardants, antioxidants, antistatic agents, optical brighteners and ultraviolet light absorbers, or ACD due to metallic fibres in a nickel-sensitized woman, have been reported.[9,10] The "nylon-dermatitis" of the 1940s was actually caused by either the dye or the finish on the fibre.[11] Sporadic cases of contact urticaria due to nylon and silk have been summarized by Hatch and Maibach.[11] As well as fibres in a strict sense, elastic ribbons of spandex and rubber used in brassières and girdles can cause allergic reactions. While fibre polymers, e.g. mercaptobenzothiazole and thiuram, have been found to cause delayed-type allergy,[11] latex predominantly causes acute-type allergy.

Finishes

Irritant and allergic reactions due to various chemical finishes such as acrylates, fire-retardants, antimicrobials and antistatic agents have been found[3–5,8,12–14] but historically most cases of allergy due to finishing agents have been caused by the formaldehyde-based resins (also called durable-press resins or permanent-press resins) that are used to impart wrinkle resistance (Table 13.1). According to Hatch and Maibach,[15] there are nine major resins used today which differ in formaldehyde-releasing potential during wear and use.[15] Urea formaldehydes such as dimethylolurea (DMU) and melamine formaldehydes (MF) such as hexamethylol melamine, which polymerize within the interstices of the fibres, and more modern resins obtained from cyclized urea derivates such as dimethylolethylene urea (DMEU) and dimethyloldihydroxyethylene urea (DMDHEU), which combine directly with the fibre,[16] have been the most common resins.

Nowadays, in the European and US textile industries, formaldehyde-based finishing agents with high rates of free formaldehyde release are substituted by

Table 13.1 Textile resin allergens[16]

Allergen	*Concentration and vehicle*
Formaldehyde	1% aq
Urea formaldehyde	10% pet
Ethylene urea	10% pet
Monomethylol urea	10% pet
Dimethylol urea	10% pet
Melamine formaldehyde	7% pet
Dimethylolpropylene urea	5% aq
Dimethylolmethoxypropylene urea	10% pet
N,N-Dimethylol-4-methoxy-5,5-dimethylpropylene urea	10% pet
Dimethyloldihydroxypropylene urea	10% pet
Dimethyloldihydroxyethylene urea	5% aq
Tetramethylolacetylene urea	5% aq

Table 13.2 Schiff's reagent method (time 15–20 min)[8]

Material needed
Fabric samples, 1 × 6cm strip
Test tubes (premarked for 5ml is helpful)
0.1N hydrochloric acid (HCl)
Schiff's aldehyde reagent (keep refrigerated)
Dropper or pipette
Water bath

Method
1. Rinse test tubes with 0.1N HCl
2. Add about 5ml of 0.1N HCl to each tube
3. Put each strip of fabric in seperate tube
4. Heat the tubes in a water bath for 5–10 min, cool tubes, then remove fabric
5. Add 5 drops of Schiff's reagent to the acid in each tube; a pink-purple (fuschia) colour indicates a positive test

agents with less free formaldehyde release. Allergy due to formaldehyde in clothing is now considerably less frequent. However, imported garments are often made from fabrics of unknown finishing technology. To determine whether the patient's material has been finished with free formaldehyde-releasing resins, the Schiff's reagent method (Table 13.2) can be used.

Having said this, formaldehyde is now accepted to be quite unreliable as an adequate screening agent for textile resin dermatitis because other formaldehyde-based finishing agents have little in the way of free formaldehyde release.[3,4,17] Clearly, a negative patch test to formaldehyde does not indicate that the patient's dermatitis is not caused by formaldehyde resins. Conversely, the relevance of a positive patch test result for formaldehyde does not suggest that clothing plays the important role in dermatitis. Nevertheless, in some cases, the causative agent is probably the resin itself or the formaldehyde that it may release.[15]

Dyes

In addition to textile resins, dyes are common causes of allergic textile dermatitis, which seems to be more frequent in women.[18] Most dyes that are reported to be responsible for textile allergy belong to the group of disperse dyes which are classified into two subgroups, azoquinone and anthraquinone dyes, and are used for dying synthetic polyester and acrylic fibres.[3,8,16,18,19] Dispers blue 106 and dispers 124 have been proved to be strong sensitizers.[19] They can disperse

Table 13.3 Textile dye allergens (Hermal)

Allergen	*Concentration and vehicle*
Disperse blue 124	1% pet
Disperse blue 1	1% pet
Disperse blue 3	1% pet
Disperse blue 106	1% pet
Disperse orange 3	1% pet
Disperse yellow 3	1% pet
Naphthol AS	1% pet
Disperse red 1	1% pet
Disperse red 17	1% pet
Disperse-mix blue	1% pet

in water and release from fibres can be increased by sweat, causing the induction and elicitation of allergic reactions. Natural fibres or mixed fibres are coloured by non-disperse azo dyes such as direct dyes, reactive dyes or acid dyes, which are less frequently associated with ACD than disperse.[20,21] Azo dyes may crossreact with paraphenylenediamine (PPD) but, according to many investigators, PPD is now accepted to be quite unreliable as a screening agent for textile dye dermatitis in general.[3,6,18,22]

Specific screening series are commercially available and include some of the well-known dye allergens (Table 13.3). However, there is an enormous number of dyes; hence, in most cases, the patient's own material should be tested.

Others

Rubber and metal materials such as nickel in garments may also cause allergic dermatitis,[10] and are discussed elsewhere (see Chapters 10 and 14).

Recommendations

In general patients, and formaldehyde-allergic patients in particular, should be advised to wash new clothing several times before wearing it, because the amount of free formaldehyde sometimes found in textiles is usually reduced effectively by washing.[3,4,8,12] Patients should be advised to avoid drip-dry or crease-resistant clothes and to use wool, nylon, polyester or acrylic fabrics, as these rarely contain significant amounts of formalin or formaldehyde resins.[23] Due to trends in fashion and leisure activity and technological developments, the patterns of textile use in clothing have changed rapidly and therefore new unknown allergens may exist. However, it is of great benefit to identify whether an allergen is a dye, a finish, etc., so that the patient can be given some general guidelines for choosing clothes.

References

1. Bendsöe N, Björnberg A, Asnes H, Itching from wool fibers in atopic dermatitis. *Contact Dermatitis* 1987; **17**:21–22.
2. Adams RM, Dermatitis due to clothing. *Cutis* 1972; **5**:577–582.
3. Cronin E, Clothing and textiles. In: Cronin E, ed. *Contact dermatitis* New York: Churchill Livingstone; 1980:36–92.
4. Sherertz EF. Clothing dermatitis: practical aspects for the clinician. *Am J Contact Dermatitis* 1993; **3**:55–64.
5. Estlander T, Jolanki R, Kanerva L, Clothing. In: Guin JD, ed. *Clothing*. New York: McGraw-Hill; 1992:297–323.
6. Seidenari S, Manzini BM, Danese P, Contact sensitization to textile dyes: description of 100 subjects. *Contact Dermatitis* 1991; **24**:253–258.
7. Estlander T, Kanerva L, Jolanki R, Occupational allergic dermatoses from textile, leather, and fur dyes. *Contact Dermatitis* 1990; **1**:13–20.
8. Storrs FJ, Dermatitis from clothing and shoes. In: Fisher AA, ed. *Contact Dermatitis*. Philadelphia: Lea & Febiger; 1986:283–337.
9. Arisu K, Hayakawa R, Ogino Y et al., Tinuvin R P in a spandex tape as a cause of clothing dermatitis. *Contact Dermatitis* 1992; **9**:324–325.
10. Hegyi E, Gasparik J, The nickel content of metallic threads in an Indian shawl. *Contact Dermatitis* 1989; **21**:107.
11. Hatch KL, Maibach HI, Textile fiber dermatitis. *Contact Dermatitis* 1985; **12**:1–11.
12. Hatch KL, Maibach HI, Textile chemical finish dermatitis. *Contact Dermatitis* 1986; **14**:1–13.
13. Andersen K, Hamann K, Cost benefit of patch testing with textile finish resins. *Contact Dermatitis* 1982; **8**:64–67.
14. Malten KE, Textile finish contact hypersensitivity. *Arch Dermatol* 1964; **89**:215–221.
15. Hatch KL, Maibach HI, Textile dermatitis: an update (I): resins, additives and fibers. *Contact Dermatitis* 1995, **32**:319–326.

16. Foussereau J, Clothing. In: Rycroft RJG, Menne T, Frosch PJ, Benezra C, eds. *Clothing*. Berlin: Springer; 1995:503–514.

17. Fowler JF Jr, Skinner SM, Belsito DV, Allergic contact dermatitis from resins in permanent press clothing: an underdiagnosed cause of generalized dermatitis. *J Am Acad Dermatol* 1992; **27**:962–968.

18. Hatch KL, Maibach HI, Textile dermatitis. A review. *J Am Acad Dermatol* 1985; **12**:1092–1097.

19. Hausen BM, Contact allergy to Disperse blue 106 and Disperse blue 124 in black "velvet" clothes. *Contact Dermatitis* 1993; **28**:169–173.

20. Seidenari S, Manzini BM, Schiavi ME, Motolese A, Prevalence of contact allergy to non-disperse azo dyes for natural fibers: a study in 1814 consecutive patients. *Contact Dermatitis* 1995; **33**:118–122.

21. Manzini BM, Motolese A, Conti A et al., Sensitization to reactive textile dyes in patients with contact dermatitis. *Contact Dermatitis* 1996; **34**:172–175.

22. Brandao FM, Hausen BM, Cross-reaction between Disperse blue dyes 106 and 124. *Contact Dermatitis* 1987; **16**:289–290.

23. Wilkinson JD, Shaw S, Contact dermatitis: allergic, clothing and shoes. In: Champion RH, Burton JL, Burns DA, Breathnach SM, eds. *Rook/Wilkinson/Ebling, Textbook of dermatology*, 6th edn. Oxford: Blackwell Science; 1998.

14. Contact Reactions to Metal Salts: Nickel Contact Dermatitis

Uta Christina Hipler and Matthias Gebhardt

Nickel sensitivity is the most common cause of allergic metal dermatitis, particularly in young women (Figure 14.1).[1] Nickel sulphate is at the top of almost any patch test result list around the world. This is due to the changes in lifestyle (increased interest in fashion and beauty, along with increased prosperity) within the latest century. Allergic reactions to fashion jewellery, brassière hooks, zippers or the metal in spectacle frames are probably the most common sources of nickel contact dermatitis. Ear-piercing commonly initiates nickel allergy earlier in life, which usually remains lifelong. The causative role of piercing for the sensitization is illustrated by the recent increase in nickel allergy in men, corresponding to the increased popularity of piercing among men. Most jewellery contains nickel; however, there is less nickel in 14 or 18 carat gold jewellery than in inexpensive fashion jewellery. Stainless steel, unless nickel-plated, will not cause an allergic reaction.

Nickel allergy may develop at any age. The true effect of the sensitization for the affected person's everyday life depends on what nickel level elicits an allergic reaction. Some people are highly allergic to nickel and may get a rash from even brief contact with nickel-containing metals, while others break out only after a long period of skin contact with nickel. This is important to consider in occupational dermatology. Many, if not most, nickel-allergic individuals can be in contact with nickel for a short period of time without problems, while a

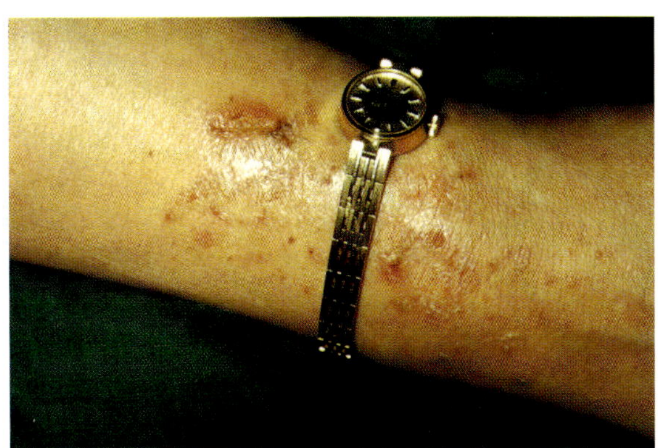

Figure 14.1: Allergic contact dermatitis due to a nickel-releasing watch.

minority can not tolerate it at all: both the individual sensitization level and the release of free nickel ions from the contact surface are factors.

Although the majority of cases are non-occupational, work-related nickel dermatitis is a predominant diagnosis in reports on permanent disability due to skin disease. Nickel dermatitis was first clinically recognized as "Das Galvanisierekzem" in Germany in 1889.[2] Occupational nickel dermatitis was common in the 1920s and 1930s,[3–5] while it was first reported in consumers in the early 1930s and later on recognized as a large-scale consumer problem in 1936.[6] The incidence of nickel sensitivity as well as the female-to-male ratio varies from one country to another and from one period of time to another, probably due to variations in the exposure to nickel. Among 5558 patients (57% females) with dermatitis who were patch tested in six Scandinavian centres, the incidence of positive reactions to $NiSO_4$ was 5.9%.[7] Incidences of 4.7–14.3% have been reported from different centres.[8] The female-to-male ratio of nickel-sensitive patients is generally high, and in six Scandinavian centres it varied from 2:1 to 15:1;[7] in Kuwait, however, the ratio was 1:3, which was due to a greater exposure of men to nickel.[9] When individuals from the general population were patch tested, in Denmark, Finland and the USA, the incidence of nickel sensitivity among women was around 10%.[10–12]

The chemistry of nickel

The brief synopsis of the chemistry of nickel provided in this chapter is condensed from several chapters by Maibach and Menné.[13] In 1751 a Swedish mineralogist, Axel Frederik Cronstedt, identified a previously unrecognized metallic element as a constituent of the common mineral *"kupfernickel"*. This mineral is now known as NiAsS (*Gersdorffite*). In Germanic folklore, nickel referred to a dwarf, devil or scamp ("Old Nick") because of the garlic odour in the copper-manufacturing process, though this was caused by the arsenic in the ore. Cronstedt named the new element "nickel" and described it as a silver-white hard, malleable, ductile metal that maintains high lustre and is a fair conductor of electricity and heat. Nickel is relatively resistant to corrosion in many acids, salts and alkaline, in fresh and salt water, and in wet and dry gases. Accounting for the widespread use of nickel are ferronickel alloys (e.g. stainless steel), cupronickel alloys (e.g. Monel metal) and precious metal alloys (e.g. German silver). The atomic number of nickel is 28 and its atomic weight is 58.71g/mol, comprising a mixture of five stable isotopes. Metallic nickel exists in two principal phases, α-nickel with a hexagonal lattice and β-nickel with a cubic lattice. The melting point of nickel is 1453°C, and the specific gravity at 25°C is 8.902g/cm^3. Oxidation states of nickel include –1, 0, +1, +2, +3 and +4, but the prevalent valences are 0 (in nickel metal and its alloys) and +2 (in most nickel salts and stable inorganic compounds). Nickel atoms contain unpaired electrons in two outer 3d orbitals and thus undergo changes in oxidation state that involve one electron. Complexion with peptides can reduce the redox potential of the Ni^{3+}/Ni^{2+} couple from 4.2V to values of 0.7–1.0V, enabling stable Ni^{3+} complexes to form under certain biological conditions.[14,15] The oxidation–reduction properties of the Ni^{3+}/Ni^{2+} couple may account for the biological roles of nickel in enzymes and coenzymes, such as ureases, dehydrogenases and factor F_{430}, which have been identified in plants and micro-organisms, and may initiate the free-radical reactions (e.g. lipid peroxidation, DNA-nucleoprotein cross-linking) that are speculated to be involved in the pathogenesis of nickel toxicity and carcinogenesis.[16]

The coordination chemistry of nickel

An excellent and extensive discussion of the coordination chemistry of nickel has been presented by Sacconi et al.[17] and more condensed summaries of nickel coordination chemistry include those of other authors.[18,19] A short overview of this topic is necessary with an emphasis on the biologically relevant chemistry. The most common geometry of nickel complexes are the 6-coordinate (octahedral), the 5-coordinate (square-pyramidal or trigonal-bipyramidal) and the 4-coordinate (square-planar or tetrahedral). Complexes containing high oxidation states of nickel (Ni^{3+}, Ni^{4+}) are generally unstable and rapidly oxidize a variety of organic compounds while forming the stable nickel(II) species. From the point of view of biochemical interest, nickel(IV) complexes have not been shown to be important. In contrast, nickel(III) species may play a biological role in genetic damage by nickel compounds, and nickel(III) states appear to be accessible to certain nickel-containing enzymes. Nickel(II) presents the most common oxidation state of nickel. A wide variety of ligands can complex with nickel(II). This element is considered to be at the borderline between hard and soft metals: it can interact with ligands that are classified as hard (water, hydroxide, ammonia, chloride, phosphate, sulphate, nitrate, carbonate), as intermediate (amines, azide, nitrite) and as soft (thiols, thiolates, CO, cyanide). An especially important ligand with regard to nickel(II) coordination is dimethylglyoxime. This ligand was first used by Tschugaeff[20] for determination of trace quantities of nickel. It forms a square-planar bis-(dimethylglyoximato) nickel(II) complex (Figure14.2) that allows for spectrophotometric or gravimetric determination of nickel in biological systems.

Several highly insoluble complexes of nickel(II) are found in the environment. For example, nickel sulphides, nickel carbonate, nickel oxide and nickel phosphate exhibit no-to-little dissolution at pH 7. Furthermore, when nickel ions in aqueous buffer are adjusted to high pH, the $Ni(OH)_2$ complex precipitates. Soluble complexes of many common organic compounds (e.g. citrate, histidine and cysteine) are also highly stable and may interfere with transport processes.

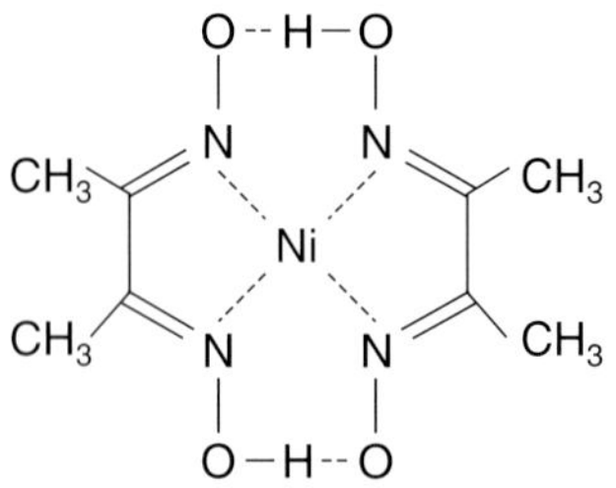

Figure 14.2: The bis-(dimethylglyoximato)nickel (II) complex.[21].

The low oxidation states of nickel (+1, 0, –1) can be found in complexes of organic compounds, especially p-acceptor ligand. From a biological perspective, however, nickel(I) complexes of tetraazamacrocycles and thiol ligands are also well known.[17] Evidence for the presence of nickel(I) in a tetrapyrrole associated with methyl coenzyme M reductase is discussed, as well as the possibility of nickel(I) in the sulphur-rich environment of the hydrogenase active site. Nickel(0) stabilization similarly requires the presence of ligands with strong p-acceptor capacity (e.g. carbonyls, phosphines, phosphites). In general, these complexes are unstable toward oxygen and water. No clear examples of nickel(0) that possess biologically relevant ligands have been described. Nickel-(–1) has been claimed to exist in several compounds, but this formal oxidation state of metal probably has little meaning. Nickel(–1) is unlikely to have any biochemical significance.

Sources of nickel exposure

Since 1940 the incidence of nickel allergy has increased considerably in parallel with the augmented use of this metal in everyday articles.[23] Today almost half the nickel production in the world is used for stainless steel, while about 10% is used in alloy steels. Cupronickel and other non-ferrous, high-nickel alloys account for 20% of the production, electroplating and certain foundry uses for 10%, and a smaller amount is used for batteries, catalysts and chemicals.

Sensitization is mainly a result of daily skin contact with corrosive metal objects containing nickel. Such everyday objects include jewellery made of German silver (containing 10–20% nickel), especially earrings for pierced ears, nickel-plated spectacle frames, buttons for blue jeans, clasps, buckles or zippers. Even jewellery of white gold with 2–15% nickel may cause eczema.[1,24,25] The amount of nickel released from such objects depends on the corrosive resistance of the object and the presence of sweat and other corrosive fluids. Owing to the chloride content and the relatively low pH, sweat may dissolve nickel. Experiments with synthetic sweat and normal saline have shown that nickel may be leached from various materials. A particular group of people called "rusters", with an abnormally high chloride concentration in their sweat, are likely to release even more nickel.[26]

An allergic patient may successfully use Fisher's dimethylglyoxime spot test to identify free nickel ions in his or her environment. One drop of a 1% solution of dimethylglyoxime in ethanol and one drop of 10% ammonia are placed on the object; the fluids are mixed and rubbed onto the object with a small cotton swab. The appearance of the red complex will indicate dissolution of nickel from the object.[1] The test is commercially available as an easy-to-use assay for the consumer in many countries. Other sources for nickel are given by occupational exposures of the skin, the oral exposure, pulmonary and iatrogenic exposures. The most relevant occupational exposure is found with electroplaters, welders and metalworkers; less with plumbers, electricians, construction workers and related trades, and much less (although regarded hazardous for nickel allergics by many physicians!) among healthcare professions and hairdressers. Episodic cases have been reported in cashiers depending on the country's coins; we have seen two patients who were not able to tolerate brief contacts with nickel coins and had to leave their jobs (Figures 14.3 to 14.5).

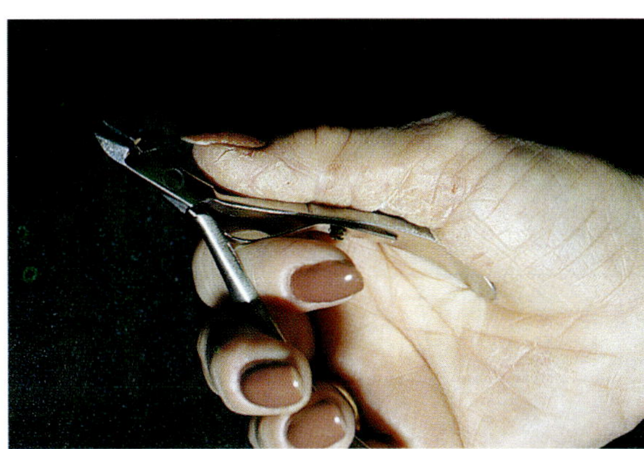

Figure 14.3: Allergic contact dermatitis to nickel.

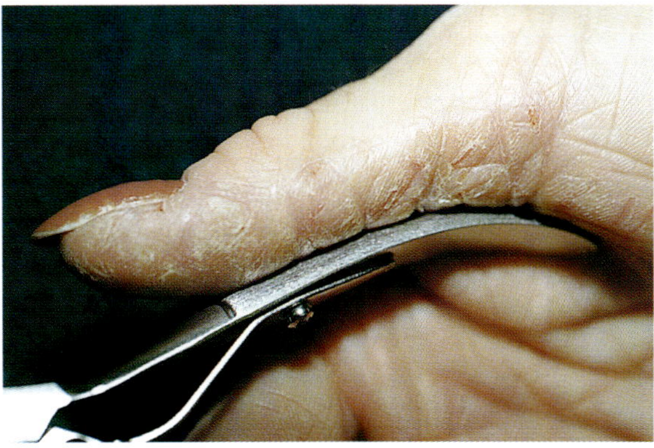

Figure 14.4: Allergic contact dermatitis to nickel.

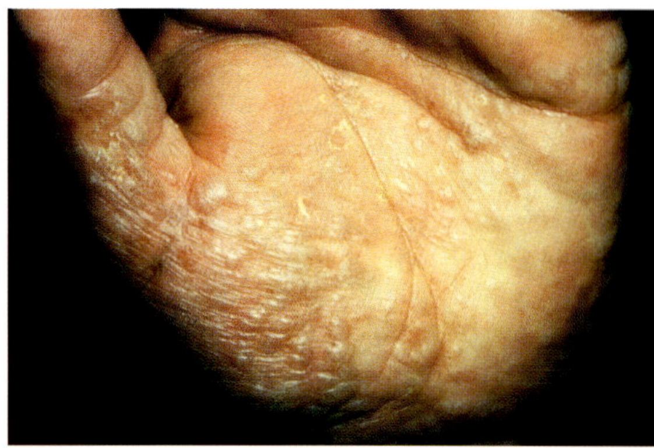

Figure 14.5: Dyshidrotic eczema (pompholyx) of the palm.

Nickel as hapten in allergic contact dermatitis

Many important contributions to the present knowledge of allergic contact dermatitis (ACD) result from studies with experimental animals, particularly mice and guinea pigs.[26] Remarkably, despite nickel being the most frequent sensitizer in humans, reproducible sensitization of guinea pigs to this allergen has met with some difficulties and no convincing sensitization of mice has been reported so far.[27] Most recent developments in the field of nickel allergy, therefore, are the result of clinical in vivo and in vitro studies.

Nickel cations, potentially generated on oxidation of metallic nickel, may readily penetrate the epidermis and associate with immunologically relevant carriers.[28] For comparison, a different situation exists for another important metal allergen, chromium: the active hapten (Cr^{3+}) poorly penetrates the epidermis but may be locally generated by reduction of readily penetrating chromate anions.[29]

In the formation of an immunogenic nickel complex at the surface of antigen-presenting cells, three possibilities exist:

- Nickel binds directly to class II molecules
- Nickel binds to other cell-membrane-associated molecules located in the close vicinity of class II molecules
- Nickel binds to soluble carrier molecules that, following uptake and eventual degradation by allergen-presenting cells, are exposed at the cell surface close to class II molecules

Recent data favour the view that direct nickel modification of class II molecules is of major importance.[30] Nickel-specific T-cell clones, derived from nickel-hypersensitive individuals, can be fully activated to proliferate and produce lymphokines in vitro in the absence of skin cells bearing class II molecules constituents, provided cells bearing class II molecules are added. Moreover, such in vitro stimulation could be obtained with serum-free culture media and chloroquine-treated allergen-presenting cells, in the absence of intracellular uptake and degradation of metal–protein complexes.[31] In line with this, Silvennoinen-Kassinen et al.[32] recently suggest that one of the two major nickel-binding proteins isolated from mononuclear cells is the β-chain of the class II molecule. Following skin contact, probably the many nickel cations that associate with other carriers either remain immunologically silent (null event) or induce suppresser cell activation (tolerance induction).

Although it cannot yet be excluded that hapten-specific T cells with the cytotoxic phenotype may contribute to contact hypersensitivity (e.g. by killing hapten-binding epidermal cells), most effector T-cells belong to the helper subclass. Obviously, in humans, no direct proof can be obtained from passive transfer experiments. The major evidence comes from in vitro studies analysing peripheral blood lymphocytes (PBL) or skin infiltrates obtained from nickel-allergic patients.[33] Using culture conditions for in vitro cloning of PBL both with helper and cytotoxic function, all the isolated nickel-specific clones were CD3+, CD4+, CD8– (T-helper–Th–phenotype).[30] This was also found for clones derived from nickel-induced skin lesions.[34]

The question as to how these cells are first activated in vivo to proliferate during primary sensitization may be answered as follows. The T-cell receptor accounts for allergen specificity through the polymorphic nature of its α and β chains. Nickel-specific T-cell receptors tend to bind to nickel-modified class II molecules, thereby allowing receptor-associated CD3 (a trimolecular complex) to provide an intracellular signal for activation. An additional signal is provided by interaction between CD2 molecules (formerly known as the sheep erythrocyte receptor) and the lymphocyte function-associated antigen 3 (LFA-3). The chance of these activation steps taking place may be further increased by other interaction molecules and their counterstructure present on Th cells and allergen-presenting cells: LFA-1/intercellular adhesion molecule 1 (ICAM-1)[35] and CD4/class II, respectively.

The direct nickel–MHC class II molecule binding on the skin antigen-presenting cells such as Langerhans cells would result in Th-cell activation. Substances such as serotonin and cytokines such as TNF-α produced by activated mast cells may increase adhesion molecule expression and thus, enhance T cell trafficking in the skin. Cytokines such as IFN-γ and interleukin-1 (IL-1) and perhaps IL-12 play a crucial role in the activation of Th1 cells. Along with possible function of CD8 cells, downregulation of nickel-induced contact dermatitis may be mediated by suppressed function of Langerhans cells via the action of activated keratinocyte-derived IL-10.[36] Despite the strong specificity of T cells imposed by their T-cell receptors, crossreactivity may be observed. A recent study using nickel-reactive T-cell clones showed donor-dependent crossreactivity with either copper or palladium (Cu at the right hand and Pd below nickel in the periodic table of the elements).[37] Cross reactivity at clonal level was never observed with other metals like cobalt and chromium. Interestingly, copper- and palladium-contact allergic reactions have been reported to occur in nickel-allergic patients almost exclusively.[38,3] During the sensitization process, proliferation of nickel-specific T cells is assumed to take place within the paracortical areas of those lymph nodes that drain the skin contact site. These conditions may be mimicked in vitro in the lymphocyte transformation test with PBLs.[40] Systemic dissemination of the resulting large numbers of nickel-specific T cells forms the basis for the development of nickel hypersensitivity. Skin hyper-reactivity to nickel may therefore be observed at all skin sites, provided that sufficient Langerhans cells are locally available.[41]

Marked preferential entry of nickel-specific T cells may occur at nickel-challenged skin sites. After sensitization, the frequency of nickel-specific T cells in the circulation is persistently increased. In addition, this frequency will show transient peaks shortly after the first and every further contact with the allergen. An inflammatory reaction therefore, when elicited within a few weeks of sensitization or boosting, will contain an increased frequency of nickel-specific T cells. Moreover, recently activated T cells possess a uniquely high migratory capacity.[42] At the skin level, selective accumulation of nickel-specific T cells at nickel-challenged skin sites may be further enhanced by two other mechanisms. First, vascular endothelial cells contain low levels of relevant interaction molecules (MHC class II, ICAM), the expression of which is increased by locally released interferon-γ.[43,44] Upon local mediator release, therefore, nickel binding to these surfaces may contribute to local adhesion and extravasation of nickel-specific cells. In support of this view, Kapsenberg et al.[34] demonstrated that approximately 10% of the T cells present at 48h in nickel-induced contact skin lesions were nickel specific. In this study, inflammatory T cells were cloned with 100% cloning efficiency, thereby providing a full reflection of the T-cell repertoire within the lesional infiltrates. As a corollary of the activation of nickel-specific T cells at a contact reaction skin site, these cells also start to proliferate. This further contributes to a strongly increased frequency of nickel-specific T cells at a nickel skin reaction site and accounts for strong and protracted eczematous reactivity as long as sufficient allergen is locally available. It should be emphasized that local frequency of specific T cells may still increase in a subsiding skin reaction despite a large fall in absolute numbers of residual T cells.[45]

The role of metal-specific T cells in this disease is well established, but the molecular interactions involved in their activation are poorly understood. Menné et al.[45] examined the T-cell receptor (TCR) repertoire in T cells activated with either $NiSO_4$ or $NiSO_4$-treated human serum albumin from allergic patients. For the three most hyper-reactive donors, a strong over-representation of the TCR BV-

17 element was found. TCR sequencing for one of these donors revealed an additional skewing for AV-1 as well as a selection for an N region encoded argine at position 95 of the BV-17 complementary determining region-3 (CDR-3). Since argine is not known to participate in nickel complexing, the suggestion is made that this selection is driven by contacts with peptide rather than nickel. However, the CDR-1 of BV-17 contains a unique combination of amino acids that bears similarities to known motifs in nickel-binding proteins or peptides. Therefore, it is proposed that the severe hypersensitivity reactions found in BV-17 overexpressors may be the result of Ni^{2+} ions bridging the germline-encoded BV-17 loop to corresponding sites in the MHC–peptide complex and thereby creating a superantigen-like enhancement of weak TCR–peptide contacts.

The recurrence of nickel hypersensitivity reactions in patients, e.g. flare-up reactions following systemic supply of nickel, can be now be well understood in the light of the above-mentioned mechanisms.

Clinical crossreactivity between metal salts

Crossreactivity phenomenon between different metal salts is a very common. Nobody knows exactly yet, if the above-mentioned immunological mechanisms are the one and only reason for it. Roughly, with a few exceptions, nickel is the allergen and the other metals are the cross reactants. Metal salts that readily crossreact with nickel include the following: cobalt (Co), palladium (Pd) and gold (Au). There is some controversy as to whether it is an immunological crossreactivity, as stated above, or a coupled sensitization based on concomittant exposure to several metals in alloys. Impurites in test materials (nickel traces in cobalt or gold salts) has been excluded by the major patch test providers. Some authors even doubt the relevance of these concomittant reactions. In contrast, one of the few and very rare single reactions to gold, palladium or cobalt without concomittant nickel allergy should always attract the attention of the dermatologist. Sources of cobalt sensitization may be found in ceramics and procelain production ("cobalt blue") and in the steel industry. Gold and palladium allergies are commonly a consequence of dental treatment, namely inlays and crowns. This question is discussed Chapter 16.

Irritant reactions of metal salts on the skin

An irritant reaction (irritant contact dermatitis – ICD) is an inflammatory reaction that is provoked by direct cell damage and not by an immune process. Characteristically the erythema is limited to the damaged contact area, the reaction area being sharp. In mild acute cases there is no itching and no oedema, papules or vesicles; the erythema appears within one day and disappears rapidly after removal of the irritatant. Some irritants can cause the skin to swell without erythema, and strong irritants can produce erosions or bullae.

Metal salts are well known to produce irritant patch test reactions, commonly of the follicular type. The test reaction is characterized by a follicular appearance of tiny papules surrounded by a normal appearing skin. The skin may be necrotic above the papules. The usual inflammatory infiltrate is lacking. However, these metal salt effects are probably more important in the artificial model of the patch test and not an everyday reality.

A very common positive-reacting non-relevant patch test allergen was cadmium chloride, which has now been withdrawn from many patch test trays due to its lack of relevance.

Prevention of nickel contact dermatitis

Immunological prevention

The more that becomes known about nickel presentation and T-effector cell function, the less we seem to know about mechanisms controlling development and expression of nickel ACD. No obvious association with HLA antigens can be detected, and development of nickel allergy may therefore primarily depend on frequency and intensity of skin contacts with the allergen.[13] Ear-piercing and use of cheap jewellery certainly represent important risk factors.[46]

In nickel allergy, no suppresser function of T cells with the suppresser/cytotoxic phenotype has been detected.[47] Nevertheless, evidence suggesting the existence in humans of afferently acting suppressor cells in nickel allergy, i.e. preventing sensitization, was obtained in an epidemiological study.[48] The frequency of nickel hypersensitivity was remarkably low in a group of junior nurses who had oral contacts with the allergen through orthodontic dental treatment.[49] Obviously, inhibition of nickel ACD can also be generated by feeding with nickel, suggesting that the induction of oral tolerance to nickel may be beneficial as an alternative immunotherapy for nickel allergy.[36]

Reducing the risk of nickel sensitization through the induction of low nickel-releasing alloys would be a primary step in the prevention of nickel allergic dermatitis in humans.

The use of binding agents and barrier creams

Over the past 40 years, several substances that chemically bind nickel have been investigated for their ability to prevent the symptoms of nickel ACD. These substances are usually incorporated into topical preparations, but oral treatments have also been used.[50] The prophylaxis with ethylene diamine tetra-acetic acid (ETD) is one of the common methods. A cream containing 15% ETD and 1% hydrocortisone reduced the allergic reaction to patch testing with 20 pence coins (16% Ni, 84% Cu) in 10 out 26 nickel-sensitive subjects challenged for 2 days.[51] Czech topical preparations containing ETD (Indulone E and Selisski ointment) delayed but did not prevent the penetration of nickel salts into damaged rabbit and human cadaver skin.[52] In a further study in nickel-sensitive subjects who where patch tested with different combinations of $NiSO_4$ and Na_2H_2EDTA, it was concluded that chelation of Ni^{2+} deactivates its antigenic ability and the topical application of an active chelating agent inhibits the appearance of a positive nickel patch test over the site.[53]

The effect of bidentate sulphur-donor ligands such as diethyldithiocarbamate (DDC) and tetraethylthiuram disulphide (TETD) on the prophylaxis of nickel dermatitis has also been studied.[54] Topically applied sodium DCC (10% in polyethylene glycol, phosphate buffered to pH7) was effective in blocking the nickel patch test reaction.

5-Chloro-7-iodoquinolin-8-ol (clioquinol) is the most effective ligand yet described for the prophylaxïs of nickel dermatitis.[51] At 2 days the allergic reaction to nickel is abolished in all cases using a vioform hydrocortisone cream containing 3% clioquinol and 1% hydrocortisone.

Preparations containing diphenylthiocarbazone, diphenylglyoxime and tartaric acid have been investigated for their ability to detoxify Ni^{2+} in vitro. The preparation with diphenylglyomime was the only one to demonstrate a positive effect.[55] Kolpakov[55] has demonstrated that a cream consisting of equal proportions of petrolatum and lanolin, which contained 1% dimethylglyoxime (DMG), delayed but did not prevent the penetration of Ni^{2+} (as 10 or 20% solutions of $NiSO_4$ and/or $NiCl_2$) into damaged skin in vitro.

Other attempts at prophylaxis have been made using barrier creams and other substances. Barrier creams are intended to act as an "invisible glove", shielding the skin from potentially harmful chemicals or radiation.[56] Almost all dermatologists feel that barrier creams are not very effective in the prevention of allergic hand dermatitis. Despite this, some investigators have examined the efficacy of barrier creams in nickel allergy, particularly in patients with hand dermatitis.[57] Two barrier creams were studied, one composed of hydrocarbons and the other of hydrocarbons, silicon and cetaceum. Both exerted an inhibiting effect on the absorption of chromium and nickel through the skin.[58]

Topical cyclosporin (5% in Unguentum Merck) inhibited the patch test responses to $NiSO_4$ in four out of 18 nickel-sensitive patients.[59,60] Dexamethasone sprayed onto the skin and onto nickel-containing articles stopped the dermatitis reaction in nickel-sensitive patients.[61] The patch test reaction to a nickel-containing coin ceased in 20 subjects and a "use" test in 37 individuals showed protection against coated nickel-plated objects. Isopropyl myristate, present in the spray, seemed to be necessary for the effect, as dexamethasone aqueous solution alone did not work.

Taken together, a ligand protecting the skin from nickel dermatitis should be non-toxic, non-irritant, non-sensitizing and not absorbed through the skin. In addition, it should form a complex with Ni^{2+} that is more stable than nickel conjugate antigen, and have more rapid complexing reaction kinetics with nickel, compared with the skin–protein–nickel complexing reaction that leads to the formation of the nickel–conjugate antigen.[50] In addition, the ligand should be dispersed in a vehicle that is suitable for cutaneous application and has a pH that favours Ni^{2+} complexing (e.g. probably <7 for basic ligands such as clioquinol). The pH ranges of the epidermis and dermis are 4.2–6.5 and 7.2–7.3, respectively.[62] Therefore, the region in which the immunological reactions occur is virtually neutral, and it may be that a ligand that complexes Ni^{2+} under such conditions is favourable, in comparison with ligands that require pH conditions for Ni^{2+} complexion that are significantly greater than or significantly less than pH7. In considering a ligand for systemic use, Maibach and Menné felt that a suitable candidate should posses a high affinity for nickel inside the body and low affinity for nickel outside the body.[13] It should also be unable to act as a lipophilic ionophor across the gastrointestinal mucosal barrier and not produce side-effects after prolonged use.

Patch tests with nickel and other metal salts

It has been mentioned above that many metal salts give rise to irritant patch test reactions. A follicular appearance can indeed be of allergic origin but usually is irritant. In Europe the 5% pet $NiSO_4$ preparation is used, while in the USA the 2.5% pet $NiSO_4$ preparation is preferred. The tendency to evoke irritant reactions is higher when applying large test chambers and when increasing the exposure up to 48h.

For medicolegal reasons it is quite important to make a statement about the sensitization level. This can easily be done by testing a $NiSO_4$ concentration range from pet 5% down to 0.005%. Individuals who still react to 0.05% or less have a high likelihood of reacting upon short time contacts to nickel or traces of nickel in gold, etc.

References

1. Fisher AA, *Contact dermatitis*, 2nd edn. Philadelphia: Lea & Febinger; 1973.

2. Blasko A, Die Berufsdermatosen der Arbeiter. Das Galvanisierekzem. *Dtsch Med Wochenschr* 1889; **15**:925.

3. Bulmer FMR, Studies in the control and treatment of "nickel rash". *J Ind Hyg Toxicol* 1926; **8**:517.

4. Jadahssohn W, Schaaf F, Über die Häufigkeit des Vorkommens von Nickelekzem. *Arch Dermatol Syphilol* 1929; **157**:572.

5. Du Bois C, La dermatite du nickel. *Schweiz Med Wochenschr* 1931; **12**:278.

6. Bonnevie A, *Aetiologie und Pathogenese der Ekzemkrankheiten*. Copenhagen: Busck; 1936.

7. Magnusson B, Blohm SG, Fregert S et al., Routine patch testing IV. Supplementary series of test substances for Scandinavian countries. *Acta Derm Venereol* 1968; **48**:110–114.

8. Fregert S, Hjorth N, Magnusson B et al., Epidemiology of contact dermatitis. *Trans St John's Hosp Derm Soc* 1969; **55**:17–35.

9. Kanan MW, Contact dermatitis in Kuwait. *J Kuwait Med Assoc* 1969; **3**:129–144.

10. Kieffer M, Nickel sensitivity: relationship between history and patch test reaction. *Contact Dermatitis* 1979; **5**:398–401.

11. Peltonen L, Nickel sensitivity in the general population. *Contact Dermatitis* 1979 **5**:27–32.

12. Prystowsky SD, Allen AM, Smith RW et al., Allergic contact hypersensitivity to nickel, neomycin, ethylendiamine, and benzocaine. Relationship between age, sex, history of exposure, and reactivity to standard patch tests and use tests in general population. *Arch Dermatol* 1979; **115**:959–962.

13. Maibach HI, Menné T, *Nickel and the skin: immunolgy and toxicology*. Boca Raton: CRC Press; 1989.

14. Nieboer E, Stetsko PI, Hin PY, Characterization of the Ni[II]/Ni[III] redox couple for the nickel[II]-complex in human serum albumin. *Ann Clin Lab Sci* 1984; **14**:409.

15. Cross JE, Hughes DM, Williams DR, Critical review of the evidence for nickel[III] in animals and man. In: Brown SS, Sunderman FW Jr, eds. *Progress in nickel toxicology*. Oxford: Blackwell Scientific; 1985:109–12.

16. Sunderman FW Jr, Lipid peroxidation as a mechanism of acute nickel toxicity. *Toxicol Environ Chem Rev* 1987; **15**:59–69.

17. Sacconi L, Mani F, Bencini A, Nickel. In: Wilkinson G, Gillard RD, McCleverty JA, eds. *Comprehensive coordination chemistry: the synthesis, reactions, properties and applications of coordination compounds*. New York: Pergamon Press; vol 5, 1987:1–347.

18. Coyle CL, Stiefel EI, The coordination chemistry of nickel: an introductory survey. In: Lancaster JR, ed. *The bioinorganic chemistry of nickel.* New York: VCH Publishers; 1988:1–28.

19. Tomlinson AAG, Nickel. *Nickel Coord Chem Rev* 1981; **37**:221–296.

20. Tschugaeff L, Determination of nickel. *Z Anorg Allg Chem* 1905; **44**:144.

21. Hausinger RP, *Biochemistry of nickel.* New York: Plenum Press; 1993.

22. Wang CP, Franco R, Moura JJ, Day EP, The nickel site in active *Desulfovibrio baculatus* [NiFeSe] hydrogenase is diamagnetic. Multifield saturation magnetization measurement of the spin state of Ni(II). *J Biol Chem* 1992; **267**:7378–7380.

23. Marcussen PV, Ecological considerations on nickel dermatitis. *Br J Ind Med* 1960; **17**:65.

24. Fischer T, Fregert S, Gruvberger B, Rystedt I, Contact sensitivity to nickel in white gold. *Contact Dermatitis* 1984; **10**:23 24.

25. Brandrup F, Schultz Larsen F, Nickel dermatitis provoked by buttons in blue jeans. *Contact Dermatitis* 1979; **5**:148–150.

26. Samitz MH, Katz SA, Scheiner DM, Lewis JE, Attempts to induce sensitization in guinea pigs with nickel complexes. *Acta Derm Venereol (Stockh)* 1975; **55**:475–80.

27. Andersen KE, Maibach HI, Guinea pig sensitization assay. In: Andersen KE, Maibach KI, eds. *Current problems in dermatology*, vol 14. Basel: S. Karger; 1985:263.

28. Sunderman FW, A review of the metabolism and toxicology of nickel. *Ann Clin Lab Sci* 1977; **7**:377.

29. Polak L, Immunology of chromium. In: Burrows D, ed. *Chromium: metabolism and toxicity*. Boca Raton: CRC Press; 1983:82.

30. Sinigaglia F, Scheidegger D, Garotta G et al., Isolation and characterization of Ni-specific T-cell clones from patients with Ni-contact dermatitis. *J Immunol* 1988; **135**:3929–32.

31. Kapsenberg ML, van der Pouw-Kraan T, Stiekema FEM et al., Direct and indirect nickel-specific stimulation of T lymphocytes from patients with allergic contact dermatitis to nickel. *Eur J Immunol* 1987; **18**:977–82.

32. Silvennoinen-Kassinen S, Jakkula H, Karvonen J, Binding of nickel to the mononuclear cells and in the serum of nickel-sensitive and healthy subjects. *Clin Exp Dermatol* 1987; **12**:265–9.

33. Silvennoinen-Kassinen S, Jakkula H, Karvonen J, Helper cells (Leu-3a+) carry the specificity of nickel sensitivity reaction in vitro in humans. *J Invest Dermatol* 1986: **86**:18–20.

34. Kapsenberg ML, Res P, Bos JD, Nickel-specific T lymphocyte clones derived from nickel-contact dermatitis lesions in man. I. Heterogeniety based on requirement of dendritic cell subsets. *Eur J Immunol* 1987; **17**:861–5.

35. Rothlein R, Dustin ML, Marlin SD, Springer TA, A human intercellular adhesion molecule (ICAM-1) distinct from LFA-1. *J Immunol* 1986; **137**:1270–74.

36. Sosroseno W, The immunology of nickel-induced allergic contact dermatitis. *Asian Pac J Allergy Immunol* 1995; **13**:173–181.

37. Scheper RJ, Von Blomberg M, Brynzeel DP, Studies of T cell fine specificity using nickel-reactive T cell clones. *J Invest Dermatol* 1986; **87**:165–71.

38. Walton S, Investigation into patch testing with copper sulphate. *Contact Dermatitis* 1983; **9**:89–90.

39. van Loon LAJ, van Elsas PW, van Joost TH, Davidson DL, Contact stomatitis and dermatitis to nickel and palladium. *Contact Dermatitis* 1984; **11**:294–7.

40. von Blomberg-van der Flier M, van der Burg CKH, Pos O et al., In vitro studies in nickel allergy: diagnostic value of dual parameter analysis. *J Invest Dermatol* 1987; **88**:362–8.

41. Asherson GL, Allwood GG, Inflammatory lymphoid cells. *Immunology* 1972; **22**:493–502.

42. van Dinther-Janssen ACHM, van Maarsseveen ACMT, de Groot J, Scheper RJ, Comparative migration of T and B lymphocyte subpopulations into skin inflammatory sites. *Immunology* 1983; **48**:519–27.

43. Wagner CR, Vetto RM, Burger DR, Expression of I-region associated antigen (Ia) and interleukin 1 by subcultured human endothelial cells. *Cell Immunol* 1985; **93**:91–104.

44. Christensen OB, Linström C, Löfberg H, Möller H, Micromorphology and specificity of orally induced flare-up reactions in nickel-sensitive patients. *Acta Derm Venereol (Stockh)* 1981; **61**:505–10.

45. Menné T, Hjorth N, Reactions from systemic exposure to contact allergens. *Semin Dermatol* 1982; **1**:15.

46. Santucci B, Nickel dermatitis from cheap earrings. *Contact Dermatitis* 1989; **21**:245–248.

47. Silvennoinen-Kassinen S, Ilonen J, Tiilikainen A, Karvonen J, Inhibition of in vitro nickel sulphate reaction by anti-HLA-DDR antisera. Lack of demonstrable suppressor cells in peripheral blood in nickel unresponsiveness in man. *J Invest Dermatol* 1981; **77**:417–20.

48. van der Burg CKH, Bruynzeel DP, Vreeburg KJJ, Hand eczema in hairdressers and nurses: a prospective study. *Contact Dermatitis* 1986; **14**:275–279.

49. Sjovall P, Christensen OB, Moller H, Oral hyposensitization in nickel allergy. *J Am Acad Dermatol* 1987; **17**:774–778.

50. Gawkrodger DJ, Healy J, Howe AM, The prevention of nickel contact dermatitis. A review of the use of binding agents and barrier creams. *Contact Dermatitis* 1995; **2**:257–265.

51. Memon AA, Molokhia MM, Friedmann PS, The inhibitory effects of topical chelating agents and antioxidants on nickel-induced hypersensitivity reactions. *J Am Acad Dermatol* 1994; **30**:560–565.

52. Resl V, Sykora J, In vitro testing of ointments designed to protect the skin from damage by chromium and nickel. *Dermatol Woschr* 1965; **151**:1327–1340.

53. Kurtin A, Orenteich N, Chelation deactivation of nickel ion in allergic eczematous sensitivity. *J Invest Dermatol* 1954; **22**:441–445.

54. Menné T, Kaaber K, Treatment of pompholyx due to nickel allergy with chelating agents. *Contact Dermatitis* 1978; **4**:289–290.

55. Kolpakov FI, The role of protective external preparations in the prevention of the penetration of chromium and nickel into the skin. *Vestn Derm I Venr* 1964; **38**:8–12.

56. Fullerton A, Menné T, In vitro and in vivo evaluation of barrier gels in nickel contact allergy. *Contact Dermatitis* 1995; **32**:39–45.

57. Hogan DJ, Dannaker CJ, Lal S, Maibach HI, An international survey on the prognosis of occupational contact dermatitis of the hands. *Derm Beruf Umwelt* 1990; **35**:143–147.

58. Starek A, Barrier creams in the prevention of occupational contact dermatitis – an experimental study. *Pol J Occup Med Environ Health* 1991; **4**:261–268.

59. Aldrige RD, Sewell HF, King G, Thomson AW, Topical cyclospirin A in nickel contact hypersensitivity: results of a preliminary clinical and immunohistochemical investigation. *Clin Exp Immunol* 1986; **66**:582–589.

60. De Rie MA, Meinardi MM, Bos JD, Lack of efficiacy of topical cyclosporin A in atopic dermatitis and allergic contact dermatitis. *Acta Derm Venereol* 1991; **71**:452–454.

61. Fisher AA, Steroid aerosol spray in contact dermatitis; prophylactic use with particular reference to nickel hypersensitivity. *Arch Dermatol* 1964; **89**:58–60.

62. D'Auria D, *Occupational health and safety open learning module HD4. Harmful dusts, gases, vapours and mists unit*. London: HMSO 1988;1–4.

15. Regional Contact Dermatitis

Andrea Bauer

Eyelid dermatitis

Diagnosis of eyelid dermatitis is often complex. Endogenous as well as exogenous factors are important. Allergic, irritant and airborne contact dermatitis are common. Maybe because of special anatomical features, e.g. the thinner epidermal layers of the eyelids, they are more easily affected by contact dermatitis than other parts of the body. This is the case even when the substances are not used directly on the eyelids, but on the scalp, face or hands, without affecting the primary site of exposure.[1] In addition to contact dermatitis, the differential diagnoses include seborrhoeic dermatitis, atopic eczema, rosacea and psoriasis. In one study,[2] Valsecchi et al. screened 1158 consecutive patients of their allergy unit from January 1990 to April 1991 for eyelid dermatitis. One hundred and fifty patients were diagnosed as having eyelid dermatitis with or without dermatitis on other parts of the body; 90% of the patients were females. The majority of cases were judged to be allergic contact dermatitis (ACD), fewer being irritant or atopic dermattis and even fewer being seborrhoeic dermatitis. The main allergens found in eyelid dermatitis patients were nickel sulphate (no relevance found), preservatives (methyl(chloro)isothiazolone, MCI/MI; diazolidinyl urea) and fragrance mix. Less important allergens were formaldehyde, balsam of Peru, potassium chromate and local antibiotics (neomycin sulphate). There was no big difference in sensitization between patients with eyelid dermatitis and patients without.

These findings are confirmed by many other studies, which also show high incidence of allergic contact dermatitis (ACD) in patients with eyelid dermatitis.[3] First-line sources of allergens are facial and eyelid cosmetics and topical drugs. Second-line sources are syndets (synthetic detergents), shampoo, make-up removers and nail varnish ingredients.

Cosmetics and cleansers

Causative ingredients in cosmetics are fragrances, preservatives/antimicrobials such as formaldehyde, MCI/MI or parabens, emulsifiers and basal ointments like stearyl alcohol and wool alcohol, toluene sulphonamide formaldehyde resin in nail varnish, sunscreens such as *p*-aminobenzoic acid derivatives and cinnamate, colophony, balsam of Peru, and surfactants such as cocamidopropyl betaine.[4,5]

Sensitization to cocamidopropyl betaine, an amphoteric surfactant, has increased in recent years. Cocamidopropyl betaine (CPB) and its intermediate dimethylaminopropylamine (which is suggested to be the major allergen) can be found in shampoos, shower gels, moisturizers, deodorants, bubble baths and contact lens fluids. Besides occupational contact dermatitis in hairdressers, CPB may be a relevant allergen in patients with cosmetic allergy, especially on the eyelids. Fowler[6] saw 5.7% positive patch test reactions to CPB in 210 patients with dermatitis of the head. One per cent aq CPB is recommended for routine testing. Nevertheless, many cases remain doubtful in terms of the relevance of CPB. Repeated open application tests (ROATs) with final products are always recommended.

Occasional cases of eyelid dermatitis due to nickel sulphate and rubber vulcanization accelerators in nickel- or rubber-plated eyelash curlers have been reported.[7,8]

Allergic eyelid dermatitis due to nail varnish is commonly caused by toluene sulphonamide formaldehyde resin.[4,9] Another allergen source in nail cosmetics is the use of artificial nails, which are fixed by methacrylate glue.

I recommend testing of the standard tray and the cosmetics tray as well as the patient's own cosmetics. "Leave-on" products – mascara, eye liners – should be tested as they are. These products do have some irritative potential. In such cases, I recommend testing single ingredients (after asking the manufacturer for details). "Rinse-off" cosmetics – shampoos, face cleansers – should be tested diluted (1% aq and 0.1% aq).

Testing on intact skin sometimes gives false-negative results in patch tests. In such cases, testing should be done on stripped skin. Performing of ROAT on the skin of the eyelids is not recommended.

Topical drugs

Sensitization to topical drugs in patients with eye diseases is an important medical problem. One has to consider not only drops and ointments topically applied on the eyes or eyelids but also transfer of topical drugs from remote sites of the body by contaminated fingers. Besides sensitization to medicaments, one has to also consider the other ingredients, such as preservatives and ointment bases. Ockenfels et al.[11] identified antibiotics, phenylephrine and thiomersal as the leading allergens in patients with ACD of the eyelids.[11]

Antibiotics and antimicrobial agents such as chloramphenicol have been reported to cause ACD.[12] Phenylephrine, a mydriatic agent, is commonly used by ophthalmologists before fundoscopic examinations. Because of its vasoconstrictive effects it is also used in nasal decongestants and in topical preparation in otology.[13] Other relevant ophthalmological decongestants are naphazoline and tetrahydrozoline. Thiomersal is a common preservative agent in eye drops. Topical antihistamines have long been thought to be potent sensitizers; most case reports were published between 1947 and 1980. However, the majority of the

Table 15.1 Topical drugs causing allergic eyelid dermatitis
Phenylephrine in eye drops[13]
β-Blockers in eye drops[15,16]
Antibiotics in eye drops[11]
Resorcinol in an ophthalmological ointment[17]
Pilocarpine[18]
Thiomerosal[11]
Chloramphenicol/thiamphenicol in eye drops[12]
Antazoline in eye drops

studies or reports are not based on valid test procedures, therefore the sensitization potential of these topical drugs is probably overestimated.[14]

There are case reports of other topical drugs acting as allergens (Table 15.1).

I recommend testing using the standard tray, ointment bases and the patient's personal topical medicaments. Topical medicaments are tested as they are (without dilution). Irritative potential has to be considered. Testing on intact skin sometimes gives false-negative results in patch tests. In this case, I recommened testing on stripped skin. Performing of ROAT on eyelid skin is not recommended.

Occupational contact dermatitis of the face and eyelids

Occupational eyelid dermatitis is rare. Especially in Jena, a centre of the optical industry, cases of occupational contact dermatitis of the face and eyelids are seen in lens preparation workers, caused by colophony rosin in lens grinding and polishing materials. A selection of published case reports is summarized in Table 15.2.

I recommend testing using the standard tray and occupational allergens from the working environment of the patient. One should not test substances when there is no knowledge concerning the toxicity or irritancy of the constituents. When toxicity is excluded, one should test diluted.

Table 15.2 Occupational allergens in eyelid dermatitis
Acrylates in dental laboratory technicians[19–21]
Carnosol in rosemary leaves extract in the food-processing industry[22]
Triglycidyl ioscyanate in colour paint factories[23]
2,3,Epoxypropyl trimethyl ammonium chloride (EPTMAC), Kathon LX, in a starch modification factory[24]

Perianal and perigenital contact dermatitis

In the perianal area irritatant contact dermatitis (ICD) is more common than ACD, but secondary sensitization has to be taken into consideration. Inadequate hygiene regimes, inflammatory bowel disease, diarrhoea, abuse of laxatives and incontinence, as well as anatomical variations like funnel-shaped anus or perianal folds, contribute to humidity in this area and can be responsible for irritant skin changes. The irritative potential of faecal enzymes (lipase, elastase, chymotrypsin, trypsin and gall acids) has been shown in skin irritation tests. Cumulative exposure to faecal enzymes in physiological concentrations over 21 days showed severe destruction of the skin barrier as well as dermatitis.[25] Bacterial and/or mycotic superinfection is a typical complication in these patients. Table 15.3 lists the allergens involved in perianogenital dermatitis.

Among 302 patients registered in the IVDK network who were patch tested because of perianal disease, vehicles, preservatives and active substances in local medicaments dominated the list. This is because in the normally long-lasting history of patients with anogenital dermatoses, usually one or sometimes several topical drugs have been applied. Looking in detail at the allergenic ingredients in external preparations, balsam of Peru was the commonest allergen followed by fragrances, reflecting their ubiquitous presence in topical preparations. Next were cinchocaine hydrochloride and benzocaine, constituents of local anaesthetic ointments or suppositories. Fewer patients were sensitized to paraphenylenedi-

Table 15.3 Allergens in perianogenital dermatitis

Ointment bases and emulsifiers	Wool alcohol
	Amerchol L 100 (indicator for wool alcohol allergy)
	Propylene glycol
	Stearyl alcohol
	Cetyl alcohol
	Propylene glycol ointment
Balsam of Peru, fragrances, propolis	
Preservatives	Kathon CG
	Parabens
	Euxyl K400 methyldibromoglutaronitrile:phenoxyethanol (4:1)
Local anaesthetics	Cinchocaine hydrochloride
	Benzocaine
Active substance	Bufexamac
	Steroids
	Antibiotics
	Compositae extracts

amine, reflecting the sensitization to *para*-group allergens such as parabens. Further relevant preservatives were MCI/MI and methyldibromoglutaronnitrile/2-phenoxyethanol. Sensitization rates to the latter have risen in recent years and are 2-4% in patients suspected to have contact allergy. The high sensitization rate is due to its common use in cosmetics and toiletries, e.g. in moistened toilet tissues. Sensitization presumably takes place due to intensive use of moistened toilet tissues. In the last few years the sensitization rate to methyldibromoglutaronnitrile/2-phenoxyethanol has approached that of MCI/MI.[26–28] Reactions to conventional toilet paper or recycled toilet paper were shown to be often irritative because of their rough texture, not because of their toxic ingredients.[29] Neomycin is the leading allergen among antibiotics and may therefore be recommended as screening substance. Compared with an aged- and sex- matched group of patients, sensitization has been found to be impressively elevated especially to balsam of Peru, cinchocaine hydrochloride, *p*-phenylenediamine, benzocaine and preservatives (Geier J and Schnuch A, pers. comm.). These allergens can be found in basic preparations, ointments containing vegetable extracts, local anaesthetic preparations (cinchocaine hydrochloride, benzocaine), steroid-containing ointments (clobetasol propionate in Dermovate), soaps, syndets, shower gels and so on. Corresponding with these data, Marren et al.[30] found topic medicaments and their constituents to be responsible for ACD in 37 out of 39 patients with anogenital dermatoses. Other relevant allergens are natural rubber latex and its ingredients (see Chapter 5) in condoms.

Studies of ACD in the perianal area in women reveal local anaesthetics to be the most important allergen, followed by antibiotics, corticosteroids and fragrances. Looking at the allergen list in combined anogenital dermatitis, antibiotics are the most common allergen followed by corticosteroids, local anaesthetics, fragrances and antiseptics.[31] In patients who have vestibulitis and vulvodynia, which are pain syndromes similar to glossodynia, patch testing is not the first-line diagnostic approach. Only in 1 of 5 patients with vestibulitis or vulvodynia was ACD described. More often, contact allergy is seen secondarily in patients who have chronic vulvar dermatoses such as lichen sclerosus, lichen planus, psoriasis or long-lasting ICD.[30] In patients who have perianal eczema, I recommend testing standard, basal ointment and anal tray. In addition, testing of the patient's own products (such as currently and formerly used medicaments), basic mild ointments and cleansers is recommended. These preparations should be tested as they are.

In the perianal area many dermatoses mimic each other. Besides ICD and ACD, one has to consider psoriasis, atopic eczema, infections (bacterial, mycotic or viral), blistering diseases, inflammatory diseases such as lichen planus, lichen sclerosus et atrophicus, adverse drug reactions, benign or malignant epithelial and adnexal tumours, and infectious diseases (see Table 15.4).

Table 15.4 Differential diagnoses of contact dermatitis in the anogenital region

Blistering diseases	Pemphigus, cicatricial pemphigoid
Infectious diseases	Candidasis, bacterial infection, human papilloma virus infection, herpes simplex infection
Allergic diseases	Protein contact dermatitis, urticaria
Primary eczema	Atopic eczema, lichen simplex, seborrhoic dermatitis
Symptomatic dermatitis	Perianal folds, haemorrhoids, fissures, fistulas, proctitis psoriasis
Inflammatory diseases	Lichen sclerosus, lichen planus
Pain syndromes	Vulvodynia, vestibulitis
Benign tumours	Hidradenoma papilliferum, cysts
Malignant tumours	Malignant melanoma, basal cell carcinoma, vulval intraepithelial neoplasia I–III
Steroid atrophy	
Vitiligo	

Foot dermatitis

Foot dermatitis is a diagnostic and therapeutic challange. As for other body sites, there are many differential diagnoses to be considered. In cases with a chronic recalcitrant course that is not responding to any therapy, one has to consider contact allergy. Allergen sources are shoes (Figure 15.1), socks, cleansers, cosmetic products, basic preparations and topical drugs.[33,34] The typical clinical feature is the involvement of all exposed areas of the feet. The dorsal aspect is the most commonly affected site, followed by the soles (Figure 15.2). Usually, the interdigital area is excluded.

Freeman[35] reported 55 patients with ACD due to their shoes. The most common allergens were rubber components, in particular rubber antioxidants

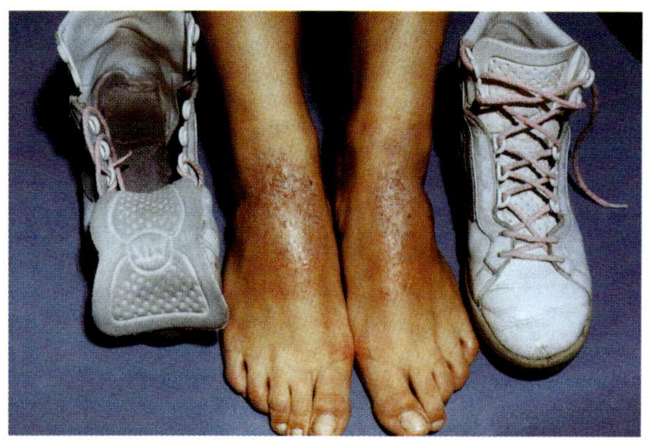

Figure 15.1: Allergic contact dermatitis to shoe material.

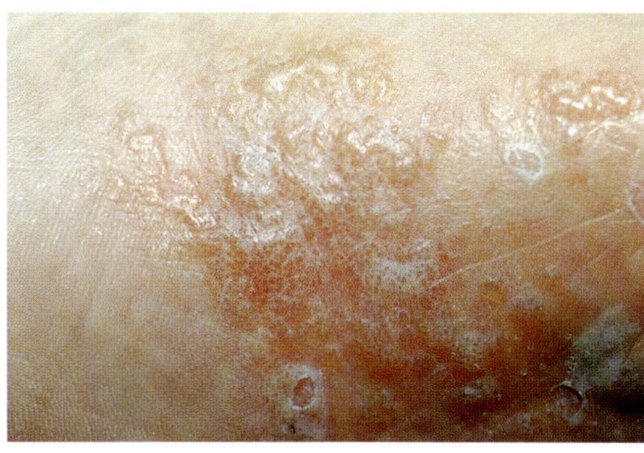

Figure 15.2: Dyshidrotic eczema of the sole.

such as mercaptobenzothiazole, followed by chromate (used as a tanning agent in the leather industry), *p*-tert-butylphenol formaldehyde resin (which is the main tackifier in adhesives in shoe linings and insoles) and colophony (used as a tackifier for heel and toe stiffeners). Thiourea (thiocarbamide), an antioxidant used in the manufacture of rubber, may also cause foot dermatitis. A less important allergen was paraphenylendiamine, a marker for allergy to *para*-group substances such as dyes and preservatives.[35] Vegetable tannings do not play a major role.[36]

Socks are able to cause contact dermatitis due to their components, such as dyes, rubber components, preservants; they are also able to act as allergen carriers. Allergens, in particular mercaptobenzothiazole from shoes, leach out from sweat-contaminated cotton socks and have been shown to cause foot dermatitis; single washing or boiling did not to do away with the contamination.[37] Supporting factors are hyperhidrosis, leaching out the allergens from socks and shoes, as well as pre-existing foot dermatitis with second-line allergy (Figure 15.3).

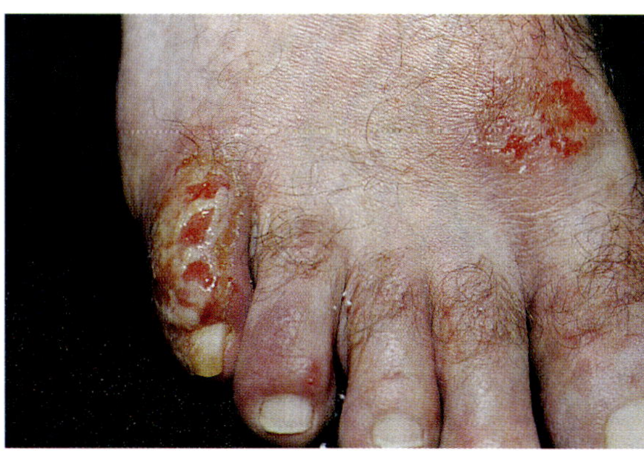

Figure 15.3: Non-specific foot dermatitis with bacterial superinfection.

I recommend patch testing using the standard tray, because most relevant allergens are represented. In addition, samples of the footwear, topical drugs and basic preparations used by the patient should be tested.

References

1. Fisher AA, Cosmetic dermatitis of the eyelids *Cutis* 1984; **34**:216–221.

2. Valsecchi R, Imberti G, Martino D, Cainelli T, Eyelid dermatitis: an evaluation of 150 patients. *Contact Dermatitis* 1992; **27**:143–147.

3. Nethercott JR, Nield G, Holness L, A review of 79 cases of eyelid dermatitis. *J Am Acad Dermatol* 1989; **21**:223–230.

4. De Groot AC, Contact allergy to cosmetics: causative ingredients. *Contact Dermatitis* 1987; **17**:26–34.

5. Ricci C, Vaccari S, Cavalli M, Vincenzi C, Contact sensitization to sunscreens. *Am J Contact Dermat* 1997; **8**:165–166.

6. Fowler JF, Cocamidopropyl betaine: the significance of positive patch test results in twelve patients. *Cutis* 1993; **52**:281–284.

7. Cabrita JC, Goncalo M, Azenha A, Goncalo S, Allergic contact dermatitis of the eyelids from rubber chemicals. *Contact Dermatitis* 1991; **24**:145–146.

8. Grandjean P, Nielsen GD, Andersen O, Human nickel exposure and chemobiokinetics In: Maibach HI, Menne T, eds. *Nickel and the skin immunology and toxicology*. Boca Raton: CRC Press; 1989:9–34.

9. Fisher AA, *Contact dermatitis*, 3rd edn. Philadelphia: Lea & Febiger; 1986:77–81, 383–385.

10. Kanerva L, Lauerma A, Estlander T et al., Occupational ACD caused by photobonded sculptured nails and a review of (meth)acrylates in nail cosmetics. *Am J Contact Dermatitis* 1996; **7**:109–115.

11. Ockenfels HM, Seemann U, Goos M, Contact allergy in patients with periorbital eczema: an analysis of allergens – data recorded by the information network of the departments of dermatology. *Dermatology* 1997; **195**:119–124.

12. Le Coz CJ, Santinelli F, Facial contact dermatitis from chloramphenicol with cross sensitivity to thiamphenicol. *Contact Dermatitis* 1998; **38**:108–109.

13. Wigger-Alberti W, Elsner P, Wüthrich B, Allergic contact dermatitis to phenylephrine. *Allergy* 1998; **53**:217–218.

14. Szolar-Platzer Ch, Maibach HI, Allergic contact dermatitis to topically applied antihistamines. *Dermatosen* 1996; **44**:205–212.

15. Labadie GF, Lepoittevin JP, Calix I, Bazex J, Contact allergy to beta-blockers in eye drops: Cross sensitivity? *Ann Dermatol Venerol* 1997; **124**:322–324.

16. Garcia F, Blanco J, Juste S et al., Contact dermatitis due to levobunolol in eyedrops. *Contact Dermatitis* 1997; **36**:230.

17. Massone L, Anonide A, Borghi S, Usiglio D, Contact dermatitis of the eyelids from resorcinol in an ophthalmic ointment. *Contact Dermatitis* 1992; **29**:49.

18. Cusano F, Luciano S, Capozzi M, Verrilli DA, Contact dermatitis from pilocarpine. *Contact Dermatitis* 1998; **29**:99.

19. Rustemeyer T, Frosch PJ, Occupational skin diseases in dental laboratory technicians. (I). Clinical picture and causative factors. *Contact Dermatitis* 1996; **34**:125–133.

20. Nethercott JR, Allergic contact dermatitis due to an epoxy acrylate. *Br J Dermatol* 1981; **4**:697–703.

21. Kanerva L, Estlander T, Jolanki R, Tarvainen K, Occupational ACD caused by exposure to acrylates during work with dental prothesis. *Contact Dermatitis* 1993; **28**:268–275.

22. Hjorther AB, Christophersen C, Hausen BM, Menne T, Occupational ACD from carnosol, a naturally-occuring compound present in rosmary. *Contact Dermatitis* 1997; **37**:99–100.

23. Wigger-Alberti W, Hofmann M, Elsner P, Allergic contact dermatitis to phenylephrine. *Am J Contact Dermat* 1997; **8**:106–107.

24. Estlander T, Jolanki R, Kanerva L, Occupational ACD from 2,3, epoxypropyl trimethyl ammonium chloride (EPTMAC) and Kathon® LX in a starch modification factory. *Contact Dermatitis* 1997; **36**:191–194.

25. Anderson PH, Bucher AP, Saeed I et al., Faecal enzymes: in vivo human skin irritation. *Contact Dermatitis* 1994; **30**:152–158.

26. De Groot AC, Van Ginkel CJ, Weijland JW, Methlydibromoglutaronitrile (Euxyl K400): an important “new” allergen in cosmetics. *J Am Acad Dermatol* 1996; **35**:743–747.

27. Van Ginkel CJ, Rundervoort GJ, Increasing incidence of contact allergy to the new preservative 1,2-dibromo-2,4-dicyanibutane (methyldibromoglutaronitrile). *Br J Dermatol* 1995; **132**:918–920.

28. Lewis FM, Shah DJ, Gawkrodger DJ, Contact sensitivity in pruritus vulvae: patch test results and clinical outcome. *Am J Contact Dermat* 1997; **8**:137–140.

29. Blecher P, Korting HC, Tolerance to different toilet paper preparations: toxicological and allergological aspects. *Dermatology* 1995; **191**:299–304.

30. Marren P, Wojnarowska F, Powell S, Allergic contact dermatitis and vulvar dermatoses. *Br J Dermatol* 1992; **126**:52–56.

31. Goldsmith PC, Rycroft RJG, White IR et al., Contact sensitivity in women with anogenital dermatoses. *Contact Dermatitis* 1997; **36**:174–175.

32. Petersen CS, Lack of contact allergy in consecutive women with vulvodynia. *Contact Dermatitis* 1997; **37**:46–47.

33. Parkinson RW, Griffin GC, Dermatitis of the feet. *Postgrad Med* 1997; **101**:95–98, 101–102, 107–110.

34. MacKenzie-Wood AR, Freeman S, Severe allergy to sorbolene cream. *Austr J Dermatol* 1997; **38**:33–34.

35. Freeman S, Shoe dermatitis. *Contact Dermatitis* 1997; **36**:247–251.

36. Bajaj AK, Gupta SC, Chatterjee AK, Singh KG, Shoe dermatitis in India. *Contact Dermatitis* 1988; **19**:372–375.

37. Rietschel RL, Role of socks in shoe dermatitis. *Arch Dermatol* 1984; **120**:398.

A. Pigatto PD, Bigardi AS, Cusano F, Contact dermatitis to cocamidopropyl betaine is caused by residual amines: relevance, clinical characteristics and a review of the literature. *Am J Contact Dermatitis* 1995; **6**:13–16.

B. De Groot AC, Van der Walle HB, Weyland JW, Contact allergy to cocamidopropyl betaine. *Contact Dermatitis* 1995; **33**:419–422.

C. Ortiz FJ, Postigo C, Ivars J et al., Allergic contact dermatitis from pilocarpin and thiomersal. *Contact Dermatitis* 1991; **25**:203–204.

16. Allergy Problems in Dentistry

Matthias Gebhardt

Dentistry is one of the most important sources of patients with dermatological allergy. This is not necessarily caused by a high incidence of allergic reactions in these patients. An exaggerated overestimation of the role of allergies to dental materials is likely to increase the number of anxious patients who are afraid of the "dangerous influence" of dental materials such as dental amalgams, filling materials, alloys and acrylic dentures. Nevertheless, there is indeed a considerable number of individuals who are affected by allergic stomatitis, cheilitis and perioral dermatitis.

Dentists, dental assistants and laboratory technicians work in an environment characterized by wet work, rich in chemical and physical irritants and possible allergens. This chapter, therefore, deals with both groups of affected people – patients and dental workers. As a rule of thumb, it is the dental technician who is most likely to develop allergies to dental materials, followed by dentists and their assistants and, last, by patients.

Allergy problems in patients

Various dental materials are included when talking about allergy problems in dentistry. Table 16.1 offers a shortened list of the different chemical classes of materials.

Dental amalgams

As has often been the case earlier this century, intolerance reactions to dental amalgams are currently a focus of interest. Toxicological reviews and studies are discussing harmful actions of amalgams and they are enthusiastically taken up by the mass media. The abundance of popular science publications in the mass media and scientific media has made patients, medical doctors and dentists feel quite uncomfortable about amalgams. In my experience, patients who ask for allergy tests to amalgam usually want a toxicological examination and not exclusion of genuine allergy. A thorough explanation may help to avoid of unnecessary patch tests to amalgam. Genuine allergic reactions seem to be rather rare, given the distribution of amalgam in the normal population.

Chemically, dental amalgams are alloys of mercury with various metals (Ag, Sn, Cu, Zn). In the dentist's surgery, prefabricated alloy powder is mixed with mercury of high purity (99.99%) in standardized quality. By diffusion, mercury enters

Table 16.1 Materials used in dentistry

Dental amalgam
Metal alloys used for inlays, crowns, bridges, partial removable dentures and orthodontic wires
- Noble metals
  - high gold content alloys
  - low gold content alloys
- Base metals
  - Ag–Pd
  - Ni–Cr
  - Cr–Co
  - Ti

Porcelain inlays, veneers and crowns
Composite fillings (resin)
Glass ionomer cement, light-curing glass ionomer cement (compomer)
Denture acrylates
Temporary fillings (zinc oxide–eugenol pastes)
Dental impression materials
Pharmaceuticals (local anaesthetics, antibiotics, antimicrobials)
Plaster

between the alloy particles, forming the plastic and, later on, the solid dental amalgam. Former amalgams were subject to the following chemical reaction:

Ag_3Sn (gamma-0-phase) + Hg $\rightarrow$ Ag_3Hg_4 (gamma-1-phase) + Sn_8Hg (gamma-2-phase).

Sn_8Hg used to be the part most susceptible to corrosion. Modern gamma-2-free amalgams are characterized by a faster binding reaction and reduced corrosion. Due to their excellent plastic features and stability, these gamma-2-free amalgams will remain the standard filling material in dentistry, at least for some years to come. Despite their improved stability, however, gamma-2-free amalgams do release very small amounts of mercury, especially in the first few days. From a toxicological point of view, mercury is mainly absorbed by inhalation or ingestion. Seafood is enriched in organic mercury components, due to water pollution. Mercury concentrations below 5µg/l blood and 5µg/l urine are generally accepted to be "normal" in most countries. Patients who have dental amalgam fillings have average concentrations of 0.7µg Hg/l in blood and up to 9µg Hg/l in urine. Negative health effects can hardly be seen below 20µg/l in blood. The World Health Organization accepts a daily uptake of approximately 40µg mercury, including alimentary intake. Approximately 20–30µg/day are attributed to alimentary factors.[1] A new amalgam filling may initially release 1–5µg/cm^2, gradually decreasing to 0.1–0.3μg/cm^2 on day 5. A steady state of approximately 0.03μg per day and per filling is usually reached later on. Mercury uptake from amalgam fillings may be increased in gum-chewers and in bruxism.[2]

The oral mucosa may be affected by amalgams in three different ways:

- Amalgam tattoos
- Oral lichen planus
- Allergic stomatitis

Amalgam tattoos

Bluish- to black-appearing pigmentation of the oral mucosa close to an amalgam filling are probably caused by traumatic implantation of small amalgam particles bursting from the high-speed drill into the surrounding mucosa. Amalgam tattoos are well-tolerated non-pathological changes that do not require diagnostic or therapeutic action, except perhaps in differential diagnosis of pigment naevi or even mucosal melanoma.

Oral lichen planus

A neighbouring amalgam filling may initiate or trigger a mucosal lichen lesion by both irritation or allergic reactions (Figure 16.1). Clearing of the lesion after amalgam removal does not definitely discriminate between allergy and irritation. Taking into consideration the high number of patients who have oral lichen planus and the low number with type IV sensitization to amalgams, irritant mechanisms are probably a more frequent cause of this mucosal disorder than are allergies. However, among patients with oral lichenoid lesions, those with a positive patch test to mercury experience more complete healing after removal of the amalgam filling than those who are patch test negative (45.2 versus

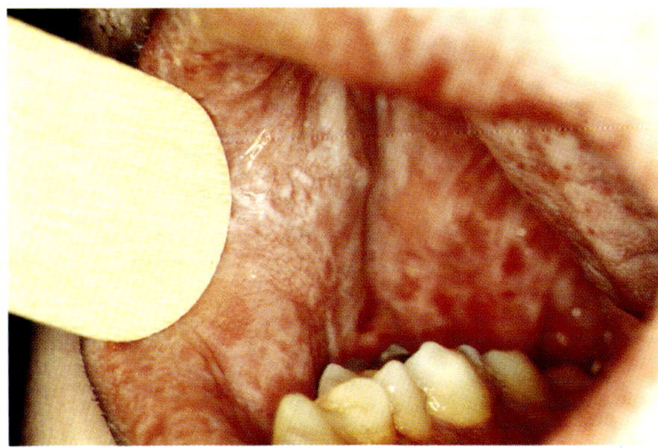

Figure 16.1: Lichenoid lesions of the oral mucosae.

20.0%).[3] A patch test with amalgam metals is in my opinion justified when oral lichen appears in a patient with amalgam fillings. Elemental and ammoniated mercury have been found to be positive more frequently in oral lichen patients whose amalgam fillings are in contact with lesions than in a reference group.[4,5] Interestingly, patch test positivity is also more pronounced in patients whose lesions contact the amalgam filling than in patients with lesions in adjacent but noncontacting areas. Some investigators recommend longer test readings, up to 10 days, because the test reaction may be lichenoid itself and slowly developing; others do not see a benefit in doing so.

Allergic stomatitis

Allergic stomatitis caused by dental amalgam is a rarity and its existence is even questioned by some authors. As mentioned above, amalgam filling material releases hardly any significant level of mercury as a consequence of superficial chemical oxidative processes. This very small amount is probably not able to induce sensitization but may rarely be able to boost or maintain pre-existing sensitization. Saliva washes away most of the mercury traces into the gastrointestinal tract. The lower number of mucosal antigen-presenting cells compared to epidermal antigen-presenting cells, together with disturbed hapten mechanisms due to the lack of stratum corneum on the musocal surface, further contribute to the improbability of the oral mucosa reacting in an allergic way.

Local toxic reactions

Some authors do also add local toxic reactions to dental amalgams to the list of possible side-effects. This type of reaction is caused by constant influence of low-concentration toxic agents such as mercury from amalgam, characterized by a clear anatomical relationship between the filling and the mucosal lesion. Because the clinical features of the lesions do not differ from allergic contact stomatitis, the diagnosis is obtained by exclusion based on a negative patch test, according to Holmstrup.[6] I would caution against making certain diagnoses such as toxic effect in this critical field of medicine. It may be difficult to explain the difference between a local toxic (or irritant?) effect of amalgam and systemic amalgam intoxication to the patient.

Non-oral problems

Interactions of amalgams with organs other than the oral mucosa are possible, in both toxic and allergic ways. Two different manifestations of amalgam allergy may occur extraorally:

- Perioral dermatitis
- Generalized eczema/exanthema

As a rule of thumb, only those reactions which are closely time-related to a dental treatment (implantation, excavation or polish of an amalgam filling) may be attributed to amalgam. The chronological relation should be in accordance with the mechanism of a type IV reaction according to Gell and Coombs (from some hours to a few days). Amalgam allergy should be self-limiting or at least self-improving because of the surface passivation.

Patch tests for amalgam sensitivity

Despite the different metals contained in dental amalgams (Hg, Cu, Sn, Ag), allergy is mainly caused by mercury. I do not recommend patch testing patients without morphological oral findings who report uncharacteristic oral phenomena such as pain, burning sensations, battery sensations or taste disturbances (Table 16.2). The inorganic mercury compound Hg (II) amide chloride, but not organic ones such as thimerosal, is considered an indicator allergen for amalgam allergy. This is very important because thimerosal reactions very often follow a "silent sensitization" by vaccinations that contain thimerosal (hepatitis, FSME (tick-borne encephalitis), influenca, diphtheria, etc.).

Epimucosatest

Optimally, all oral lesions suspected to be allergic should be tested by application of test materials to the reacting tissue, the oral mucosa. Until now, this procedure has been disappointing because of difficulties in devising and manufacturing an application device. The device would have to be well fitting and non-irritant to the application site. It would be necessary to make a device for each individual patient. All efforts to establish such a diagnostic tool have been single attempts without standardization. There are no defined morphological test reading criteria for +, ++, +++ and irritation. Another controversial point is

Table 16.2 Indications for a patch test to amalgam

1. Oral lichen planus (in close anatomical relation to an amalgam filling)
2. Perioral dermatitis in a patient with amalgam inlays
3. Generalized exanthema/eczema (systemic contact dermatitis)

(2) and (3) show deterioration after seeing a dentist and fade away within 2 or 3 weeks

the test concentration, which should probably be higher than on the back; some authors recommend a 5–10 times higher concentration; again there are no controlled studies to define these parameters.

What to do in proven amalgam allergy

If a single case of genuine amalgam allergy, mostly due to mercury, has been discovered then the fillings should be removed step by step but not at all once, because the release of the allergen is most pronounced during removal procedures. A latex rubber dam may protect the patient against ingestion or inhalation of mercury vapour during treatment.

This book does not deal with toxicological procedures and mechanisms concerning amalgam but the allergist is confronted with that problem very often, therefore I would like to briefly give my opinion about this problem. Whenever mercury intoxication is being considered, the level of release of mercury into urine and its content in blood may be helpful for diagnosis. In order to mobilize mercury depots from parenchymatous organs (despite normal range mercury in blood or urine), the chelant 2,3-dimercaptol-propansulphonic acid (DMPS) has been extensively used. The increase following intravenous DMPS is related to the organ concentrations of that metal. It is important to collect 24h urine but not the artificial peak concentration that occurs 30 min after intravenous application of DMPS. I refer the patient to an environmental toxicologist when such an assay is required.

There certainly is a correlation between the number of amalgam inlays and the increase in urine mercury after DMPS. Conversely there is a close relation of spontaneous mercury elimination and depot concentrations, therefore the DMPS assay might be of no value. Detection of oral currents between metallic inlays are not helpful in my opinion. The same is true for electroacupuncture, according to Voll, which is quite well accepted among dentists in complementary medicine. Detection of mercury levels in saliva, e.g. after chewing gum, are also favoured by some dentists. However, different individual saliva amounts release tiny metallic parts of amalgam (which can not be resorbed) and the lack of a relationship between levels of saliva mercury and absorbed mercury are just a few facts illustrating why saliva tests are avoidable and are not recommended in my experience.

According to a recent review on dental materials,[7] none of the assumed hazardous effects of dental amalgams on the brain, kidneys and immune system have been proved in scientific studies.

Dental alloys

Crowns, bridges, inlays, onlays and orthodontic appliances are made of dental alloys. Noble metal alloys consist of gold, palladium and smaller amounts of iridium, ruthenium, silver and platinum. They are known to be biocompatible, on the basis of toxicological examination. Base metal alloys have gained widespread usage due to their lower cost and better mechanical properties.[8] While gold, silver, aluminium and base metal alloys have been used in the past for the fabrication of dental appliances, more and more warnings against one or the other metal have been published on the grounds of toxicity and allergy. Indeed, patients who claim various subjective symptoms related to dental restoration materials have a significantly higher frequency of patch test positivity for nickel sulphate, potassium dichromate, cobalt chloride, palladium chloride and gold sodium thiosulphate than do eczema patients.[9] However, the clinical relevance of these reactions has to be questioned.

Palladium allergies are usually associated with nickel sensitization. Most individuals who react to palladium are primarily sensitized to nickel and only crossreact to palladium.[10,11] The rate of crossreactivity between nickel and palladium depends on the induction level, i.e. patients reacting to serial dilution of nickel are more likely to crossreact.[12] Moreover, the rate of patch test reactivity to palladium and cobalt significantly increases with the strength of the test reactions.[13] Crossreactivity seems to occur on a T-cell clonal level and is not due to concomitant natural exposure to both metals.[14] In a study among Finnish schoolchildren receiving orthodontic treatment, Kanerva et al.[15] found a much higher frequency of allergic patch test reactions to palladium chloride in girls than in boys (11 versus 1%). This difference was attributed to the differing frequency of ear-piercing in the two groups, not to orthodontic metal exposure. All except 3 of the 48 positive palladium reactions were accompanied by an allergic patch test reaction to nickel sulphate. This is in agreement with others who have found that isolated palladium allergies are quite uncommon. Therefore, there has been much discussion whether to palladium allergies are relevant. Furthermore, in spite of the potential adverse biological effects of palladium ions, the risk of using palladium in dental casting alloys appears to be extremely low because of the low dissolution rate of palladium ions from these alloys.[16] I recommend avoiding palladium use in palladium-allergic patients but not forcing the dentist to remove all palladium-based alloys when a contact allergy to this metal is diagnosed but no clinical signs are obvious.

From the prosthodontist's point of view it is not only the sum of several chemical elements but also the specific composition which makes a material corrosive and riskful for the allergic. So, many gold alloys are very corrosion resistant in contrast to silver. As a rule of thumb, noble metal alloys are more corrosion resistant than base alloys.[17] The search for the optimal intraoral metal alloy still continues. Titanium has gained some attention because of low allergenic risks, high biocompatibility and reasonable prices.[18] However, due to its high melting point, other elements such as cobalt or nickel are commonly added to improve its castability. Moreover, titanium alloys may corrode on contact with high copper amalgams and topical fluorides.[7] Thus titanium is not the best alternative for any purpose. Others alloys, such as beryllium alloys, have been seen as possible allergens too.[19]

Mode of allergy testing

Another point of controversy is the mode of allergy testing. Epicutaneous tests with metallic disks consisting of the dental alloy usually fail in patients reacting to the metal salts.[10,20] As mentioned above, it would be helpful to have a test method that is easy to use, reliable, reproducible and mimicks reality. Unfortunately, the epimucosatest is still far away from being a good alternative to well-developed, standardized, easy-to-use patch tests. Recently, the memory lymphocyte immunostimulation assay (MELISA) was introduced on the market for in vitro diagnosis of metal allergies.[21] Unfortunately, in its current form, this assay has a very low specificity compared with the patch test. It can not be recommended for diagnostic use in the detection of contact allergies.[22]

For more information see Chapter 14.

Dental acrylates

Denture-related complaints

Several symptoms may arise from introducing partial or complete removable dentures into the mouth. Most of all, ill-fitting dentures are a common cause of pain, burning, stinging or discomfort. Dentures usually become necessary later in life, in the same period many disorders appear for the first time in the life and further increase the patient's likelihood to develop denture-induced symptoms. Diabetes mellitus type II is a good example to illustrate this hypothesis. The diabetic condition increases susceptibility to moniliasis, a fungal disease further exacerbated by the mucosal microlesions induced by the solid and rough denture surface. Diabetic polyneuropathy changes the sensory reception of the mucosal nerves. Psychological changes typical in middle age (depression, phobia, etc.) decrease mental tolerance of pain. Wound-healing disturbances contribute to chronicity of mucosal lesions. All these factors may solely or in combination explain the complex aetiology of denture-induced dysaethesia. Therefore, allergic sensitization is only one of several factors possibly responsible for denture-related complaints. In my own experience it is one of the less important factors compared with other factors.

Denture material chemistry

The aim of this chapter is to give advice for dealing with patients referred to the allergist for work-up of denture stomatitis. Initially, I would like to emphasize denture material chemistry.

Complete dentures are made from methacrylates in which the teeth are imbedded. Partial removable dentures consist of both cast metal alloys and acrylic components, which hold the teeth. Since its introduction in 1937, polymethyl methacrylate (PMMA) has been the material of choice among acrylic denture base materials. The acrylic bases of dentures are made of liquid methyl methacrylate (MMA) monomers that are mixed with PMMA powder to polymerize. Various glycol dimethacrylates are introduced into the polymerization process in order to form cross-linking inter-chain bridges. The monomer liquid also contains hydroquinone, usually, to inhibit spontaneous polymerization. Benzoyl peroxide is added to the PMMA powder as initiator of the polymerization process. Alternatively, heat is applied in order to initiate the polymerization. Chemical activators such as *N,N*-dimethyl-*p*-toluidine may be used instead of heat in order start the polymerization. Recent developments have been increased based on UV- or visible light-curable acrylates (see later). These techniques require UV absorbers as ingredients of the polymerization mass.

Pigments made of cadmium might have been responsible for a few allergic reactions previously, but today cadmium is banned for toxicological and cancerogenic reasons and no longer used by producers of denture material. Light-cured acrylic dentures have been made of urethane dimethacrylate with camphoroquinone as photoinitiator.[23]

There is still some discussion whether a significant amount of residual monomer is retained after polymerization. It is generally accepted that self-curing acrylic dentures contain a greater amount of free residual monomer. Taking into consideration the fact that only the acrylic monomer (not the polymer) is capable of allergic sensitization or elicitation, it is very likely that a given content of residual monomer is responsible for a few true allergic and irritant mucosal reactions to acrylic dentures. The optimal polymerization process is the one that ensures biocompatibility of the denture; it depends on temperature, the time-course of the curing cycle and thickness of the material applied.

In contrast to silicone-based, vinyl copolymer and polyphosphazine-type chemical alternatives, soft lining materials used in prosthodontics may also contain acrylates.[7]

Evaluation of patients

What can be done for patients who come in for evaluation of their denture complaints? First of all the clinical situation should be carefully recorded and a dentist/prosthodontist should be consulted for the optimization of the prosthesis, when necessary. The patient should be advised to remove the denture overnight to reduce the exposure time to the possible allergen, traumatizing agent and *Candida*-loaded denture. Cleansing measures for the denture should be optimized as well.

If there is normal-appearing mucosa beneath the prosthesis upon repeated examination, there is no need for allergy examination at all! However, if mucosal inflammation is seen, a search for *Candida* and a topical treatment approach are justified. If these fail, a causative role for *Candida* is unlikely. If the history reveals manifestation of the condition shortly after or immediately upon the introduction of a new denture (after a previous denture has been tolerated well), if the erythema is most pronounced in the contact area and if the inflammation fades within a few days of avoidance, contact allergy may be taken into consideration. Patch testing can be done with a denture material series as recommended in Chapter 21. Metals (in partial dentures), acrylates and polymerization additives should optimally be tested after consultation of the dental laboratory technician who manufactured the denture. I want to emphasize that not only a new denture but also a repaired broken denture can be a hazard for the allergic patient, because the probability of remaining methacrylate monomers is highest in these conditions.

The testing of scrapings or filings from denture surfaces is not recommended because of the possible irritant effects of the particles.

Dental composites

Dental composites or resins are modern plastic filling materials which harden on visible or UV light. They were introduced in the early 1970s. Composites are of special interest for use in frontal teeth because of their tooth-identical colour. They are widely used as a substitute for amalgam. The material is less stable than metal inlays. Polymerization shrinkage increases the risk of dental decay progression on the margins. Because composites combine epoxy, methacrylate and peroxide groups, they are allergenic. Both the dentist and the patient come in contact with uncured monomers, which may be harmful in sensitization and elicitation of the allergic reaction. Apart from dental fillings, tooth-fissure sealing, resin-bonded bridges and crowns, and fixing of orthodontic materials to the enamel are uses for dental composite resins.

Recent developments in the field of glass ionomer cements lead to the introduction of light-curing resin-modified glass ionomer cements in 1991. Differentiation between these and classic glass ionomer cements is important in terms of resin exposure, which is only relevant in the new cements. In other words, patients who are allergic to acrylic resins will tolerate classic glass ionomer cements. The organic matrix of the composite consists of a monomer mixture (dimethacrylate), an initiator, accelerator (*N,N*-dimethyl-*p*-toluidine or 4-tolyldiethanolamine) and stabilizer. Benzophenone, benzotriazole, salicylate and resorcinol are used as UV absorbers.[24] Unwanted effects on the

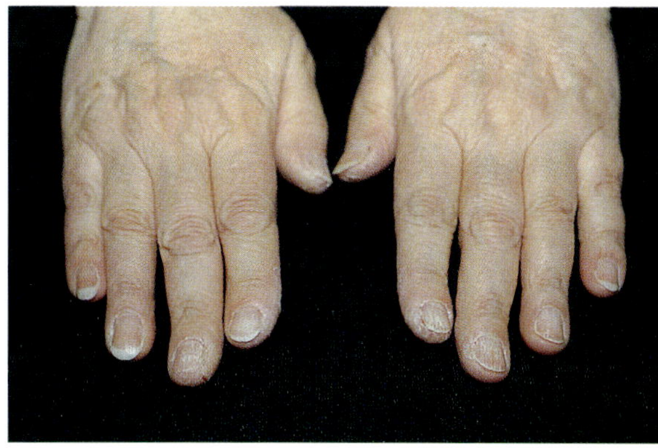

Figure 16.2: Chronic allergic contact dermatitis of the fingertips and periungual region.

pulpa–dentin system are exerted by the irritant properties of acrylics. A biocompatible base or liner is set to protect the vital tissue. 2-HEMA (2-hydroxymethyl methacrylate) is part of many dentine primers. BIS-GMA (bisphenol A glycidyl methacrylate), TEGDMA (triethylene glycol dimethacrylate) and EGDMA (ethylene glycol dimethacrylate) are common ingredients in light-curable dental fillings. Bisphenol A and epoxy resin are likely to cross react. Therefore, reactions to epoxy resin (Figure 16.2) might indicate BIS-GMA allergy in dentists, patients who have side-effects or dental personnel.

Oral care products

Although toothpaste is frequently used by almost all people in industrialized countries not too much is known about allergic reactions to toothpastes. This is particularly interesting because toothpastes contain rather common contact allergens such as essential oils, pigments and preservatives. A comprehensive list of possible ingredients and their role as allergens is given by Sainio and Kanerva.[25] Problems arise when patch testing the paste is taken into consideration. Whereas the possible allergens, e.g. flavourings, might be highly diluted within the paste, the surfactant substances are irritant to the skin and mucosa. Therefore, these cleaners make it difficult to patch test relevant allergens in appropriate concentrations. Single ingredient testing is recommendable, if the manufacturer is co-operative and will provide separate ingredients. Fluorides are very weak sensitizers, although irrelevant pustular patch test reactions are quite common.[26] Table 16.3 gives a list of possible allergenic components in toothpastes.

The same as for toothpastes can be said for mouthwashes and dentifrices. These may cause stomatitis and cheilitis or circumoral dermatitis. Because of the different sensitivity of the oral mucosa and the skin it is more likely that a person will get perioral dermatitis than stomatitis from an allergy to oral care products. Due to the nature of the products, all oral care products should be tested only

Table 16.3 Allergenic ingredients of toothpastes. Adapted and extended from Sainio and Kanerva[25] and Rietschel and Fowler[27]

Essential oils, flavourings	Peppermint, menthol, anise, cinnamic aldehyde, eugenol
Preservatives	Benzoates, thiazolinones, benzyl alcohol
Colourings	Azulene
Binding agents	Xanthan gum, agar agar
Antiseptics	Triclosan, allantoin, benzalconium chloride
Other plant substances	Tea tree oil, myrrh extract

when diluted with water or other vehicles. From a practical point of view, 1% aq may give a generally acceptable test concentration for most of the products; however, controls are strictly required when the relevance of the reaction is doubtful.

Occupational allergic contact dermatitis

When discussing occupational skin diseases in dentistry it is very important to recognize the high degree of specialization in this field. Exposure is different for orthodontists, periodontologists, prosthodontists, endodontists and general dentists. Dental technicians may be employed in large laboratories where they exclusively do plaster, metallic or acrylic work. Depending on the exposure one has to decide whether or not to use particular test trays.

The dentist and her or his team are exposed to the same dental materials as the patient. In contrast to the patient, they have repeated contact to reacting chemicals, whereas the patient has contact only for minutes (until the reaction is finished). As an example, dental composites are highly reactive epoxyacrylates but only when they have not been UV cured. The modelling of these composites brings the dentist in contact with the material if the skin is not protected by gloves. Therefore, the incidence of true allergic reactions in dentistry is much higher for occupationally exposed professionals than for patients. This is especially true for dental laboratory technicians who manufacture dentures, crowns, bridges and, not least, have intense contact with irritants. Irritant contact dermatitis in dental technicians is due to three main factors:

- Dust
- Wet work
- Chemical irritation

Dust is almost unavoidable when polishing acrylic prostheses, metallic or ceramic crowns and veneers. Face shieldings and suction devices have reduced the dust load in modern laboratories but they are too expensive for one-person laboratories, which are not uncommonly associated with a dentist's practice. Plaster dust is another common factor irritating the skin by drying out the epidermis (due to its hygroscopic capacity) and by abrasive effects from tiny plaster particles. Wet work irritation may occur in manufacturing plaster models or just in the cleaning of the hands. Chemical irritants are solvents and acrylate monomers which, apart from their allergenic capacity, are also medium-to-strong irritants to the skin. Special hazards for dental technicians are the highly reactive (meth)acrylates used to make plastic dentures or to repair broken dentures. These monomers are medium-to-strong sensitizers and therefore important occupational allergens for this profession. MMA is less sensitizing than the other new acrylic substances but, because of its wide distribution in dental materials, it remains an important occupational allergen. In addition, it has irritant properties, disturbing the epidermal barrier and thereby facilitating the sensitization of the skin. Rustemayer and Frosch[28] found MMA, 2-HEMA and EGDMA to be the major allergenic acrylate substances among dental technicians. In their 10-year statistical evaluation of the methacrylate series, Kanerva et al.[29] found 2-HEMA among the top three acrylate allergens. They further proposed six acrylates to screen for when suspecting contact allergy in dental personnel (Table 16.4).

Rustemayer and Frosch[28] and Kanerva et al.[29] pay attention to the increasing use of more and more chemical derivatives of already existing methacrylates. Therefore, current test recommendations should be discussed again from time to time, and tests should be done using the patient's own substances. Crossreactivity and concomitant sensitization are likely between the various dental acrylates. 2-HEMA is highly crossreactive with 2-HPMA (hydroxy propyl methacrylate) and EGDMA; MMA seems to be a cross reactant too.[28] Whereas the dental technician has skin contact with acrylates when manufacturing or repairing dentures (Figures 16.3 and 16.4), the dentist and her or his assistant are exposed when setting composite fillings, sealing teeth or fixing orthodontic appliances. The

Table 16.4 Acrylate screening for dental personnel

Methyl methacrylate
2-HEMA
EGDMA
TREGDMA
BIS-GMA
Urethan acrylate

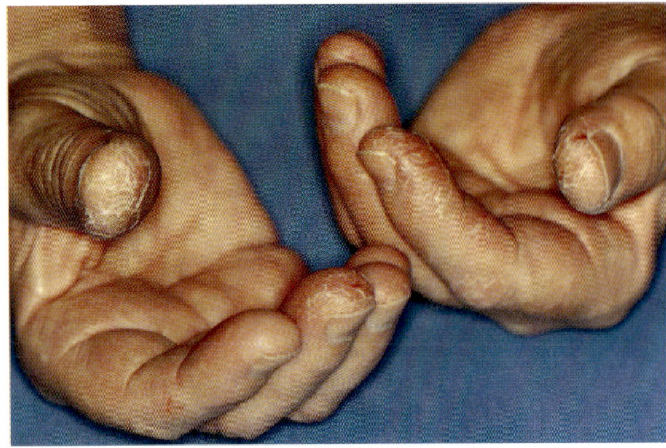

Figure 16.3: Chronic CD of the fingertips of a dental technician.

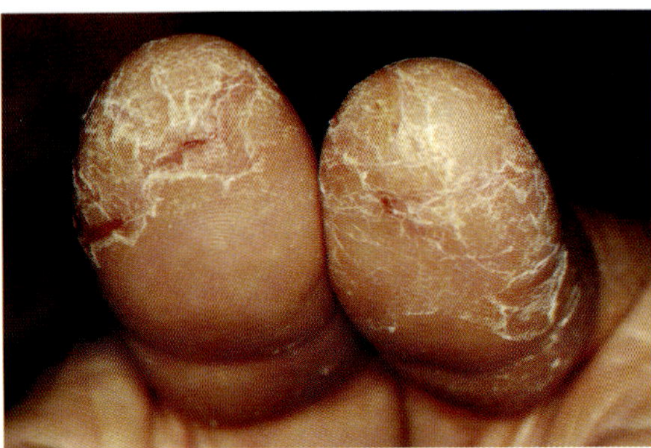

Figure 16.4: Detail of chronic CD of the fingertips.

higher incidence of occupation-related acrylate allergy among Polish dentists was attributed to the fact that they used to manufacture dentures themselves and were therefore comparable to dental technicians to some extent.[30]

Former classic occupational allergens in dentistry such as mercury from amalgam are less important today because the closed systems used in amalgam preparation now prevent release of mercury vapour into the dentist's office. However, not all dental teams have access to modern hygiene measures against mercrury, such as high-volume aspirators during cutting of an amalgam filling.[31] Contact dermatitis due to mercury exposure is much more likely in dentists than in patients when appropriate protective equipment is lacking.

Essential oils have to be considered as possible occupational allergens. Zinc oxide–eugenol pastes are commonly used as a temporary filling material. Eugenol should always be included in a dental patch test tray, for both patients and dental personnel. Eugenol and colophony have been used for periodontological dressings. Both well-known allergens may affect the dentist as well as the patient.

Table 16.5 How to deal with suspected occupational contact dermatitis in dental personnel

1. Ask about specific occupational exposure
2. Ask about pre-existing conditions (skin atopy, pre-occupational hand or flexural dermatitis)
3. Improve skin protection and skin care
4. Test disinfectants, including those from the workplace, in appropriate concentrations
5. Check for glove-induced contact urticaria/protein contact dermatitis to natural rubber latex and contact allergy to rubber chemicals
6. Consider metals in dental technicians and orthodontists/prosthodontists
7. Look for allergy to dental mercuric amalgam in dentists and assistants
8. Screen for acrylic plastics in dentists, dental assistants and technicians
9. Carefully consider relevance for positive standard allergens (colophony, epoxy resin, etc.)
10. Instruct the patient to substitute suspected dental materials and avoid hazardous work for a while

Allergic contact eczema has been attributed to the catalyst methyldichlorobenzene sulphonate in impression materials such as Impregnum.[32] Methyl-*p*-toluene sulphonate is the allergenic ingredient of Scutan, which is used as sealant for tooth and material for temporary bridges and crowns.[33]

General guidelines on dealing with suspected occupational contact dermatitis in dental personnnel are given in Table 16.5.

References

1. Hörstedt-Bindslev P, Magos L, Holmstrup P et al., *Dental Amalgam – a health hazard?* Copenhagen: Munksgaard; 1991.

2. Isacsson G, Barregard L, Selden A, Bodin L, Impact of nocturnal bruxism on mercury uptake from dental amalgams. *Eur J Oral Sci* 1997; **105**:251–257.

3. Laine J, Kalimo K, Forssell H, Happonen RP, Contact allergy to dental restorative materials in patients with oral lichenoid lesions. *Contact Dermatitis* 1992; **36**:141–146.

4. Mobacken H, Hersle K, Sloberg K, Thilander H, Oral lichen planus: hypersensitivity to dental restorative material. *Contact Dermatitis* 1984; **10**:11–15.

5. Lundstrom IMC, Allergy and corrosion of dental materials in patients with oral lichen planus. *Int J Oral Surg* 1984; **13**:16–24.

6. Holmstrup P, Oral mucosa and skin reactions related to amalgam. *Adv Dental Res* 1994; **6**:120–124.

7. Lloyd CH, Scrimgeour SN, Dental materials: 1995 literature review. *J Dent* 1997; **25**:173–208.

8. Gettleman L, Noble alloys in dentistry. *Curr Opin Dent* 1991; **1**:218–221.

9. Marcusson JA, Contact allergies to nickel sulfate, gold sodium thiosulfate and palladium chloride in patients claiming side-effects from dental alloy components. *Contact Dermatitis* 1996; **34**:320–323.

10. de Fine Olivarius F, Menne T, Contact dermatitis from metallic palladium in patients reacting to palladium chloride. *Contact Dermatitis* 1992; **27**:71–73.

11. Santucci B, Cannistraci C, Cristaudo A, Picardo M, Multiple sensitivities to transition metals: the nickel palladium reactions. *Contact Dermatitis* 1996; **35**:283–286.

12. Uter W, Fuchs T, Hausser M, Ippen H, Patch test results with serial dilutions of nickel sulfate (with and without detergent), palladium chloride, and nickel and palladium metal plates. *Contact Dermatitis* 1995; **32**:135–142.

13. Brasch J, Geier J, Patch test results in schoolchildren. *Contact Dermatitis* 1997; **37**:286–293.

14. Pistoor FH, Kapsenberg ML, Bos JD et al., Cross-reactivity of human nickel-reactive T-lymphocyte clones with copper and palladium. *J Invest Dermatol* 1995; **105**:92–95.

15. Kanerva L, Kerosuo H, Kullaa A, Kerosuo E, Allergic patch test reactions to palladium chloride in schoolchildren. *Contact Dermatitis* 1996; **34**:39–42.

16. Wataha JC, Hanks CT, Biological effects of palladium and risk of using palladium in dental casting alloys. *J Oral Rehabil* 1996; **23**:309–320.

17. Canay S, Oktemer M, In vitro corrosion behavior of 13 prosthodontic alloys. *Quintessence Int* 1992; **23**:279–287.

18. Phoenix RD, Denture base materials. *Dental Clin North Am* 1996; **40**:113–120.

19. Haberman AL, Pratt M, Storrs FJ, Contact dermatitis from beryllium in dental alloys. *Contact Dermatitis* 1993; **28**:157–162.

20. Todd DJ, Burrows D, Patch testing with pure palladium metal in patients with sensitivity to palladium chloride. *Contact Dermatitis* 1992; **26**:327–331.

21. Stejskal VDM, Cederbrant K, Lindvall A, Forsbeck M, MELISA – an in vitro tool for the study of metal allergy. *Toxic In Vitro* 1994; **8**:991–1000.

22. Cederbrant K, Hultman P, Marcusson JA, Tibbling L, In vitro lymphocyte proliferation as compared to patch test using gold, palladium and nickel. *Int Arch Allergy Immunol* 1997; **112**:212–217.

23. Ogle RE, Sorensen SE, Lewis EA, A new visible light-cured resin system applied to removable prosthodontics. *J Prosthet Dent* 1986; **56**:497–506.

24. Kanerva L, Estlander T, Jolanki R, Tarvainen K, Occupational allergic contact dermatitis caused by exposure to acrylates during work with dental prostheses. *Contact Dermatitis* 1993; **28**:268–275.

25. Sainio EL, Kanerva L, Contact allergens in toothpastes and a review of their hypersensitivity. *Contact Dermatitis* 1995; **33**:100–105.

26. Rietschel RL, Fowler JF, *Fisher's Contact Dermatitis*, 4th edn. Baltimore: Williams & Wilkins; 1995:889–892.

27. Ophaswongse S, Maibach HI, Allergic contact cheilitis. *Contact Dermatitis* 1995; **33**:365–370.

28. Rustemayer T, Frosch PJ, Occupational skin diseases in dental laboratory technicians. *Contact Dermatitis* 1996; **34**:125–133.

29. Kanerva L, Jolanki R, Estlander T, 10 years of patch testing with the methacrylate series. *Contact Dermatitis* 1997; **37**:255–258.

30. Kiec-Swierczynska M, Occupational allergic contact dermatitis due to acrylates in Lodz. *Contact Dermatitis* 1996; **34**:419–422.

31. Pohl L, Bergman N, The dentist's exposure to elemental mercury vapour during clinical work with amalgam. *Acta Odont Scand* 1995; **53**:44–48.

32. Groeningen G, Nater JP, Reactions to dental impression materials. *Contact Dermatitis* 1975; **1**:373–376.

33. Kulenkamp D, Hausen BM, Schulz KH, Kontaktallergie durch neuartige, zahnärztlich verwendete Abdruckmaterialien. *Hautarzt* 1977; **28**:353–358.

17. Allergy to Plants, Woods and Plant Extracts

Matthias Gebhardt

This chapter covers a broad range of possible botanical reasons for contact allergy. Flowers, weeds, trees (wood) and lichens are obvious causes but products made from those plants should not be forgotten. Contact allergy induced by plant products may be elicited by cosmetics, topical and systemic drugs, and food intake. Airborne contact dermatitis induced by pollens, e.g. from ragweed, is probably rather common but often not diagnosed because it mimics atopic dermatitis or chronic actinic dermatitis. Phytophotodermatitis of both toxic and allergic nature has been reported following contact with plants. A "false plant allergy" may be caused by contact with the remains of pesticides on plants. One major indicator of plant-induced allergy is the dependence of the skin complaint on growth periods of the plants, which lead to seasonal flares. Reading of the excellent papers, reviews and books written by Hausen about this topic is highly recommended to those who are more interested. Mitchell & Rook's *Botanical Dermatology* was one of the most outstanding textbooks about that particular topic. It was last published in 1979 and, fortunately, is now available on the worldwide web in a revised version by Schmidt (see Chapter 22).

Occupational dermatoses of florists, gardeners, tobacco workers, cooks, cosmetic artists, pharmacists, timber workers, etc., are frequently attributed to plants. Flower shop workers are exposed to flower work to varying degrees. Flower designers and greenhouse workers are subject to skin hazards from cutting, trimming and repotting plants in a more intense manner than wholesale persons. This distribution is in accordance with self-reported hand dermatitis in a survey among floral workers.[1] Flowers that may cause ACD have been detected among the Compositae (chrysanthemum, gerbera), Liliaceae (tulips!), Alstroemeriaceae and Caryophyllaceae (carnation) families of plants.[2] Table 17.1 lists factors that should be considered when testing flower shop workers for occupational allergy. Irritant (ICD) but not allergic contact dermatitis (ACD) seems to be the most common nature of skin complaints in occupationally exposed individuals, as Bruynzeel et al.[3] has shown for bulb growers. Even in cases of ACD among these people, pesticides turn out to be more common sensitizers than plants, which is probably due to the industrial setting in which bulbs are grown in The Netherlands. Table 17.2 gives recommendations of pesticides to be tested in floral workers.[4] Irritant exposure makes floristry a profession less suitable for skin atopics.

Table 17.1 Allergens and irritants in floral shop workers (according to Adams[5])

Plants and plant parts
Pesticides/herbicides
Fertilizers
Plant parasites
Wet work
Mechanical irritation
Soaps and detergents
Irritant plant parts

Table 17.2 Selected pesticides reported as possible causes of plant-related dermatitis

Pesticide	*Function*
Dithiocarbamates	
Maneb	Fungicide
Zineb	Fungicide
Mancozeb (contains maneb)	Fungicide
Tetramethyl thiuram disulphide	Fungicide
Barban	Herbicide
Benomyl	Fungicide and insecticide; weak sensitizer
Thiophthalmides	
Captan	Fungicide
Difolatan (Captafol)	Fungicide; not in use anymore
Folpet	Fungicide
Fluazinam	Fungicide used in Dutch tulip bulb industry
Bupirimate	Fungicide
Dyrene	Fungicide
Iodopropynyl butylcarbamate	Wood fungicide, preservative in cosmetics
Alachlor	Herbicide
Dichlorvos	Insecticide

Toxicodendron species

Probably the best-known plant-induced dermatitis is ACD from toxicodendron species such as poison ivy (Figures 17.1 to 17.3), poison oak and poison sumac, plants widely distributed in Northern America. Sensitization rates have been estimated to be up to 50–75% in the USA, with less frequent rates in urban areas.[6] Patch testing is not justified in those cases because exposure, history and distribution of dermatitis are usually self-explanatory. Poison ivy, oak and sumac

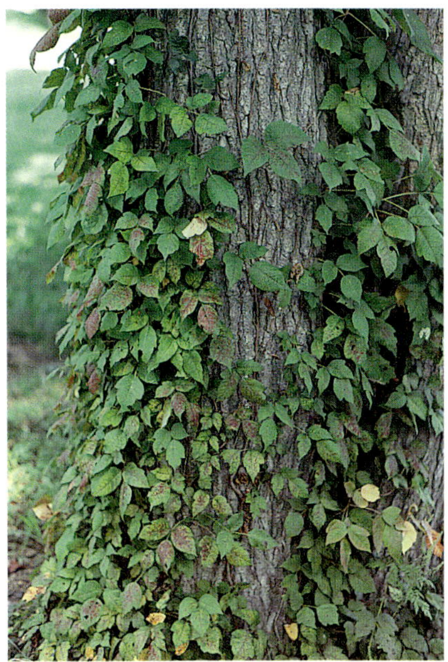

Figure 17.1: Poison ivy.

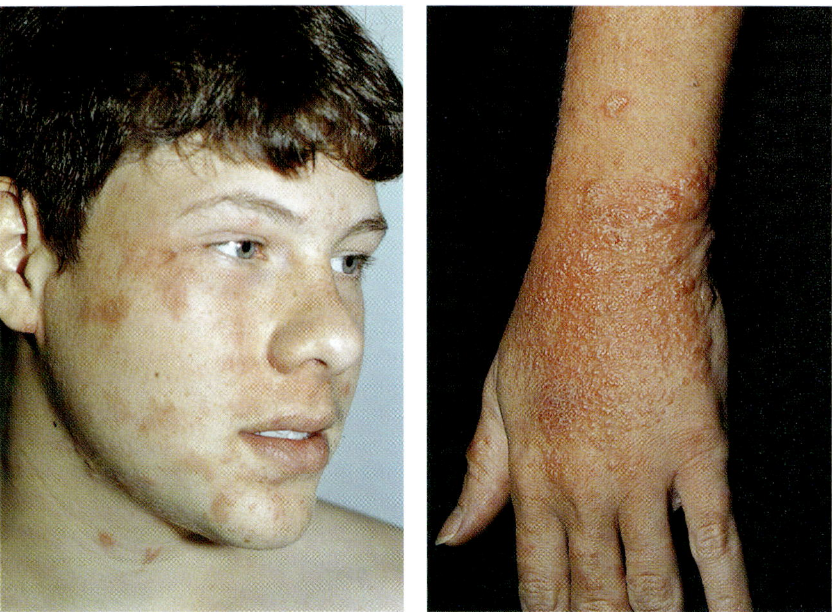

Figure 17.2 and 17.3: Allergic contact dermatitis of the face and the hand to poison ivy.

contain urushiols, the allergenic components, in the oily plant sap. Touching uninjured parts of the plant when walking by is usually non-hazardous. In contrast, brushing up against damaged plant parts or breaking plants releases the sap, which may then contact the skin and induce contact allergy. It is very hard to remove urushiol from the skin, probably due to reaction with skin proteins. Clothing or shoes may be contaminated by the oil and release small amounts over long periods, thereby maintaining skin problems. A rare cause of systemic elicitation is burning the plants and inhaling of the smoke. Much effort has been put into a reduction of the distribution of naturally occurring toxicodendron species. This should be done in the close environment of those affected by urushiol allergy. A barrier lotion (IvyBlock) containing quaternium-18 bentonite is effective in preventing ACD to poison ivy and oak.[7]

Colophony rosin

One of the plant allergens that is most important due to the distribution of its products is colophony rosin, which is a naturally occurring rosin from trees. Chemical variations have been tried to obtain a more stable raw material. Many new compounds have been developed from colophony rosin, with higher allergenicity in some compounds. Abietic acid, also available as test allergen, and especially its oxidative derivatives are the causative allergenic ingredients.[8,9] The widespread use of colophony in paper, adhesives, paints, varnishes, printing inks, plasticizers, cosmetics and drugs makes this substance one of the most important allergens on any general allergy list.[10] Colophony is an occupational allergen: classical occupational relevance is found in electronics (solder flux) and the paper and wood industries. Laminates, surface coatings for paper and other articles, are made of chemically modified rosin and may therefore also give rise to colophony contact allergy. Airborne contact dermatitis due to sawdust from coniferous woods, especially pines, red cedar and silky oak, has been attributed to colophony.[11–13] Sawdust should be patch tested along with colophony rosin to prove occupational relevance. Workers who are exposed to paints and varnishes during manufacture or use of these chemicals are also likely to get occupational contact dermatitis due to rosin. In medicine, it occurs in many types of adhesives used for tapes, bandages, hydrocolloid and surgical dressings, dental cements, periodontal dressings and wart removers.[8,14]

Turpentine oil

Turpentine oil is also a product of pine wood. It is used as solvent in paints, lacquers and varnishes. Though earlier thought to be a disappearing allergen, its frequency of test positivity has recently been increasing again.

Balsam of Peru

Balsam of Peru is an aromatic liquid smelling of vanilla or cinnamon. Intense cross reactions with fragrances are explainable by ingredients such as cinnamic acid, cinnamic alcohol, cinnamic aldehyde, vanillin, eugenol, isoeugenol and methyl cinnamate. Further information about balsam of Peru is given in Chapter 12. Some medical preparations still contain balsam of Peru as a promoter of wound healing. It has been used for skin care of the breasts in nursing women because of its antimicrobial effects. Cross reactions to spices, orange peel and cola or other soft drink may occur. Therefore, sensitization to balsam of Peru is responsible for some systemic flares of contact dermatitis following ingestion of such cross reactants. Myroxylon pereirae is the new INCI name of balsam of Peru; this may cause trouble for patients or doctors who try to identify the compound on the labelling of cosmetics.[15]

Tea tree oil

Originally grown in Australia, the tea tree (*Melaleuca alternifolia*) is currently spreading to other climatic zones of the world, such as southern Europe. Tea tree oil is increasingly used in industrial nations by consumers of complementary medicine. Indeed, it has a benefit in the treatment of inflammatory skin diseases and wound healing because of its antimicrobial effects, probably similar to those of balsam of Peru. Its use in "green" cosmetics and body-care products continues to increase. Ointments, creams, lotions, lip balms, deodorants, shampoos, soaps, even toothpastes and mouth washes may contain tea tree oil. From the legal point of view, tea tree oil is not regarded as a pharmaceutical, therefore oil of very differing qualities is available on the market. Contact dermatitis from tea tree oil is much more common than one would have expected in the light of its weak sensitizing capacity. In fact the presence of irritant, in addition to allergic reactions, is the explanation for the rather high frequency.

There is still some controversy about the allergenic compounds in tea tree oil. Eucalyptol (1,8-cineol) was first described to be the major allergen.[16] Others have not confirmed the allergenicity of eucalyptol.[17] Possible allergenic components include *p*-cymen, D-limonene, α-terpinene, aromadendrene, terpinen-4-ol and α-phellandrene.[17] Summarizing the recent studies, D-limonen, α-terpinene and aromadendrene seem to be the relevant allergens, whereas *p*-cymen and eucalyptol are not of importance.[18]

For patch tests consider using older, oxidized preparations of the oil, because their capacity to elicit skin reactions seems to be much higher than of fresh oil, which will hardly ever give a positive result. According to BM Hausen (pers.

comm.), the fresh oil can be artificially aged by leaving it exposed to the air, sunlight and room temperatures in a clear glass bottle for a couple of days. Afterwards, the dilution chosen for patch test purposes depends on the time of incubation, the general rule of the older the oil, the higher the dilution.

Propolis

Not unlike the "tea tree oil" problem is propolis. In nature, it is collected by honey bees as a resin from poplar buds and less commonly from other trees, depending on the individual environment. It is increasingly used in "green" cosmetics and medications for topical and systemic use. As for tea tree oil, propolis has some antimicrobial and anti-inflammatory effects, which makes it suitable for treatment of wounds, inflammatory skin diseases and systemic inflammatory diseases. The major allergenic components, caffeic acid and its derivatives (1,1-dimethylallyl caffeic acid ester, 3-methyl-2-butenyl caffeate, phenylethyl caffeate), are mostly strong sensitizers. A few other substances are regarded as medium-to-low sensitizers. Propolis has 13 constituents in common with balsam of Peru, therefore both are cross allergenic.[19]

Compositae

The Compositae are one of the largest groups of plants in the world with thousands of species. They occur frequently in our natural environment, as deliberately cultivated plants and as weeds. Ragweed is of special interest because its allergen is in its pollen and is therefore distributed by air currents, causing airborne contact dermatitis. Some species and their sensitizing capacity are shown in Table 17.3. Despite a low sensitizing capacity, lettuce was among the common compositae allergens in a recent Danish study on greenhouse workers.[20] Seasonal localized eczema, one year suddenly turning into widespread dermatitis, indicates Compositae dermatitis.[21] Whereas, sap contact is required for elicitation and sensitization by some species (e.g. dandelion), airborne contact dermatitis is possible in other species of Compositae (e.g. ragweed). When there is particular interest in a specific plant as a possible allergen, a patch test with 1% of a 1 min ether extract in petrolatum is usually sufficient to elicit a positive patch test reaction.

Sesquiterpene lactones are generally accepted as screening allergens for Compositae sensitization. The mix consists of alantolacotone, dehydrocostus lactone and costunolide. The content of sesquiterpene lactones is responsible for a high rate of cross sensitivity between the different species of Compositae. However, in the detection of plant allergy, a Compositae plant mixture extract

Table 17.3 Sensitizing capacity of several compositae

Plant	*Sensitizing capacity*
Arnica	Strong
Artichoke	Medium
Chrysanthemum	Strong
Camomile	Medium–low
Chicory	Low
Coltsfoot	Low
Cornflower	Very low
Dahlia	?
Dandelion	Low
Feverfew	Strong
Golden rod	Low
Lettuce	Low
Marguerite	Strong
Marigold	Low
Mugwort	Very low
Ragweed	Low
Sunflower	Medium
Tansy	Medium low

of arnica, German camomile, feverfew, tansy and yarrow has been proved superior to the sesquiterpene lactone mix because the former contains other constituents (e.g. polyacetylenes, thiophenes) that may also contribute to the acquired hypersensitivity.[22] A recent Danish study failed to show a supplementary effect for the detection of Compositae allergics when including parthenolide 0.1% as a screening in addition to SL mix.[23] Tests with single species may indicate to some extent the cause of sensitization. Whereas arnica and camomile are indicators of sensitization by cosmetics and topical drugs, tansy, yarrow and feverfew are more associated with a clinical picture of airborne contact dermatitis.

Several diseases may be mimicked by compositae dermatitis. Patients who have seasonal (summer) flares of an atopic dermatitis (AD) appearance but with low serum IgE may have Compositae dermatitis. The sesquiterpene lactone mix and colophony resin have been found positive in a high percentage (36% and 20% respectively) of patients suffering from a chronic actinic dermatitis picture as well.[24] These patients were also characterized by enhanced photosensitivity to UVA and B light. Therefore, it is recommended to test for (photo)contact sensitization to these plant derived substances. Systemic contact-type dermatitis has been reported as a result of eating lettuce or laurel, both plants containing sesquiterpene lactones, or drinking herbal teas.[25,26] Taken together, Compositae dermatitis is easily overlooked. In my opinion, a screening allergen should be routinely included in standard series. Sesquiterpene lactone mix 0.1% is commercially available and should be preferred in routine patch test screening for suspected Compositae allergy because of the risk of active sensitization to native plant material. It is important to note that some of the Compositae allergen preparations by Trolab/Hermal contain the emulgator sorbitan sesquioleat, which is an allergen itself. If the sensitization has been found accidentally and seems to be irrelevant, consider sorbitan sesquioleat to be the real allergen.

Tulips

"Tulip finger", a common occupational ACD of tulip farmers, is caused by the ingredient tuliposide A occurring in tulips, lilacs and related flowers. Contact with bulbs is especially harmful.[27] A chronic craqueling eczematous reaction of the fingertips is the characteristic clinical appearance. The same picture based

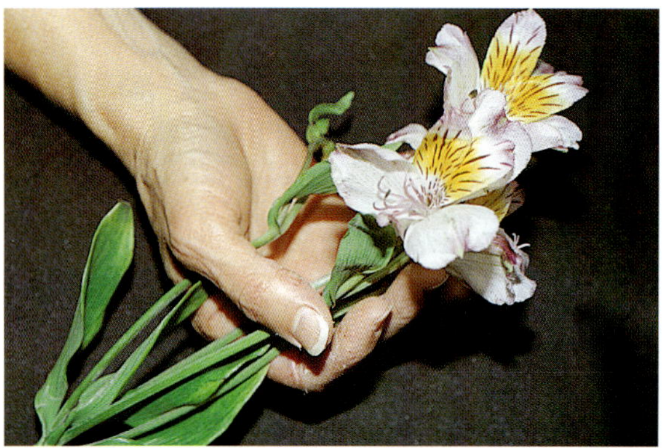

Figure 17.4: Occupational ACD to *Alstromeria* in a florist.

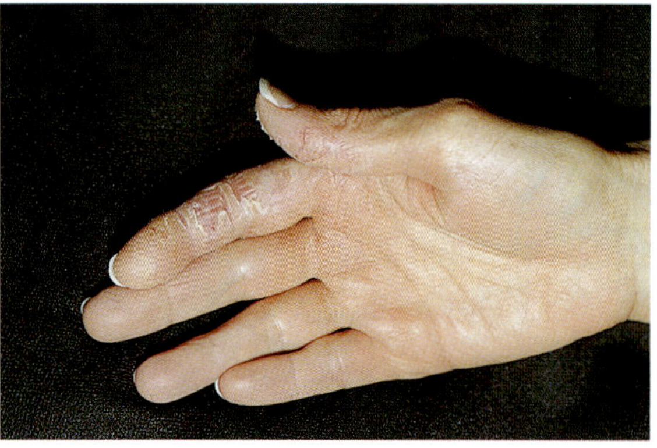

Figure 17.5: Occupational ACD to *Alstromeria* in a florist.

on the same allergens (tuliposides A and B) may be caused by *Alstroemeria* species, with the Inka lily as the best known example. This flower, belonging to the Amaryllidaceae family, is another common sensitizer among florists and flower growers (Figures 17.4 and 17.5) due to the increasing popularity of this decorative plant. Tuliposide A from *Alstroemeria* species has been found to be responsible for occupation-related skin disease of florists in approximately one-third of tested individuals.[1,28] In non-occupational patients it is less important.

Other plants and plant products

Primula allergy is not infrequent in patients who are occupationally exposed to these flowers, and it also occurs accidentally. Although patch testing with plant material is recommended in some reviews of the topic,[29] I disagree and warn against testing native material from those plants. The allergen responsible is primin, which is 2-methoxy-6-n-pentyl-4-benzoquinone.

Henna is used as alternative for chemicals in hair dying. The preparation is made from leaves of *Lawsonia intermis*, a plant grown in Asiatic and North American countries. Airways allergies and immediate-type skin reactions have been attributed to it.[30] Reports of ACD have been less common.[31] Concentrations of 10% pet have been used for patch test purposes.

Another source of occupational contact dermatitis is **Frullania**, a lichen containing sesquiterpene lactones. It grows on trees, on the ground or even on rocks and is one of the possible causes of "wood cutters disease", an eczema mainly affecting the free areas of the body (face, neck and hands).

Chemotechnique provides a **wood mix**, consisting of pine, spruce, birch and teak, which are commonly used in furniture production.

Wood tar mix, containing tars of pine, beech, juniper and birch, is available for further division of tar allergies into single wood tar components. One has to take into consideration that tars are mixtures of multiple constituents. Therefore, the quality of various tar preparations is a crucial problem with test preparations and final products, depending on the purification steps used and the source of the tar.

ICD may arise from plants that have small spines, e.g. cacti. Chemical irritation due to ingredients such as capsaicin in hot peppers is another source of eczema induction.[32] However, common plant families such as Compositae, Primulaceae, Araceae (*Dieffenbachia*), Euphorbiaceae (Christmas star), Araliaceae (ivy) and Geraniaceae were reported for occupational ICD in a Danish survey among gardeners and greenhouse workers.[33] Many plants are irritant when occluded in a patch test for 1 or 2 days. Whenever a patch test reaction to a native part of a plant occurs, one should consecutively patch test sufficient controls to exclude irritancy caused by the test.

In addition to contact dermatitis, there are also a few cases of IgE-mediated contact urticaria, asthma and rhinitis/conjunctivitis to flowers. In a recent report from The Netherlands, de Jong et al.[34] found mugwort, sodilago and *Alstroemeria* pollen to be good screening allergens for immediate-type allergy to flowers. Similar to contact dermatitis, there was a strong cross sensitization between the Compositae family plants.

Phytophotodermatitis

Phytophotodermatitis is a condition characterized by a burning painful eruption of blisters on erythematous skin, leaving long-lasting striate hyperpigmentation. It occurs frequently after contact to plant sap psoralens and other phototoxic plant agents belonging to the furocumarins or anthraquinones. UV exposure on a sunny day is required as an essential co-factor; moisture is another common attributing factor. Patch testing or photo patch testing is not justified because the clinical picture is highly characteristic. Moreover, there is no sensitization to the phototoxic agents, except in a few cases who are also allergic to the phototoxic substances. Plants commonly involved are *Heracleum* species, parsnip, celery, angelica, scabwort, pelea, lime and *Ficus* plants.[35] Skin protection by gloves and protective clothing is a strict requirement for working on a sunny day with plants well-known for their phototoxic capacity.

Summary

Table 17.4 summarizes factors that should prompt suspicion of a plant allergy. The approach to testing is is outlined in Table 17.5.

Table 17.4 When to suspect plant allergy
Seasonal flares of eczematous eruptions
Atopic dermatitis without IgE or typical history
Chronic actinic dermatitis pattern
Sun-induced dermatitis
Use of "green" cosmetics or drugs
Occupational exposure to plants and plant products
Systemic contact dermatitis associated with food or drugs

Table 17.5 What to test if plant allergy is suspected

1. Products made of plants
   Preserve the original of the product, if possible, together with the ingredient list.
2. Plants:
   First determine the family or species of the plant which is likely to cause the problem. Test with commercial plant allergens if available. Do not test native material of *Primula, Alstroemeria*, lilies, onion, garlic, iris, hyacinth, daffodils, croton sap, poison ivy/oak and Christmas star sap. Otherwise, patch native plant parts for no longer than 24h. Squeezed plant sap is less irritant than plant parts in terms of mechanical irritation. A dilution series using water and ethanol is recommended. False-negative reactions are much less common than false positive, irritant test reactions.
3. If no particular plant is under suspicion
   Screen with sesquiterpene lactone mix, fragrance mix, colophony (abietic acid), usninic acid, primin, tuliposide. Consider pesticides.

References

1. Thiboutot DM, Hamory BH, Marks JG, Dermatoses among floral shop workers. *J Am Acad Dermatol* 1990; **22**:54–58.
2. Lamminpää A, Estlander T, Jolanki R, Kanerva L, Occupational allergic contact dermatitis caused by decorative plants. *Contact Dermatitis* 1996; **34**:330–335.
3. Bruynzeel DP, de Boer EM, Brouwer EJ et al., Dermatitis in bulb growers. *Contact Dermatitis* 1993; **29**:11–15.
4. Hogan DJ, Pesticides and other agricultural chemicals. In: Adams RM, ed. *Occupational skin disease*, 2nd edn. Philadelphia: WB Saunders; 1990:547–577.
5. Adams RM, *Occupational skin disease*, 2nd edn. Philadelphia: WB Saunders; 1990:622–623.
6. Baer RL, Poison Ivy Dermatitis. *Cutis* 1986; **37**:434–436.
7. Marks LG, Fowler JF, Sherertz EF, Rietschel RL, Prevention of poison ivy and poison oak allergic contact dermatitis by quaternium-18 bentonite. *J Am Acad Dermatol* 1995; **33**:212–216.
8. Guin JD, Colophony (Rosin). In: Guin JD, ed. *Practical contact dermatitis*. New York: McGraw-Hill Inc; 1995:115–124.
9. Hausen BM. *Allergiepflanzen – Pflanzenallergene.* Landsberg: Ecomed; 1988.

10. Sadhra S, Foulds IS, Gray CN et al., Colophony uses, health effects, airborne measurement and analysis. *Ann Occup Hyg* 1994; **38**:385–396.

11. Cook DK, Freeman S, Allergic contact dermatitis to multiple sawdust allergens. *Aust J Dermatol* 1997; **38**:77–79.

12. Meding B, Ahman M, Karlberg AT, Skin symptoms and contact allergy in woodwork teachers. *Contact Dermatitis* 1996; **34**:185–190.

13. Watsky KL, Airborne allergic contact dermatitis from pine dust. *Am J Contact Dermatitis* 1997; **8**:118–120.

14. Sasseville D, Tennstedt D, Lachapelle JM, Allergic contact dermatitis from hydrocolloid dressings. *Am J Contact Dermatitis* 1997; **8**:236–238.

15. de Groot AC, Weyland JW, Conversion of common names of cosmetic allergens to the INCI nomenclature. *Contact Dermatitis* 1997; **37**:145–150.

16. de Groot AC, Weyland JW, Systemic contact dermatitis from tea tree oil. *Contact Dermatitis* 1992; **27**:279–280.

17. Knight TE, Hausen BM, *Melaleuca* oil (tea tree oil) dermatitis. *J Am Acad Dermatol* 1994; **30**:423–427.

18. Beckmann B, Ippen H, Teebaum-Öl. *Dermatosen* 1998; **46**:120–124.

19. Hausen BM, Evers P, Stuwe HT et al., Propolis allergy. Studies with further sensitizers from propolis and constituents common to propolis, poplar buds and balsam of Peru. *Contact Dermatitis* 1992; **26**:34–44.

20. Paulsen E, Søgaard J, Andersen KE, Occupational dermatitis in Danish gardeners and greenhouse workers (III). *Contact Dermatitis* 1998; **38**:140–146.

21. Paulsen E, Andersen KE, Compositae dermatitis in a Danish dermatology department in 1 year (II). Clinical features in patients with compositae contact allergy. *Contact Dermatitis* 1993; **29**:195–201.

22. Hausen BM, A 6-year experience with compositae mix. *Am J Contact Dermatitis* 1996; **7**:94–99.

23. Orion E, Paulsen E, Andersen KE, Menne T, Comparison of simultaneous patch testing with parthenolide and sesquiterpene lacton mix. *Contact Dermatitis* 1998; **38**:207–208.

24. Menage H duP, Ross JS, Norris PG et al., Contact and photocontact sensitization in chronic actinic dermatitis: sesquiterpen lactone mix is an important allergen. *Br J Dermatol* 1995; **132**:543–547.

25. Dooms-Goossens A, Dubelloy R, Degreef H, Contact and systemic contact-type dermatitis to spices. *Dermatol Clin* 1990; **8**:89–93.

26. Veien NK, Ingested food in systemic allergic contact dermatitis. *Clin Dermatol* 1997; **15**:547–555.

27. Gette MT, Marks JE, Tulip fingers. *Arch Dermatol* 1990; **126**:203–205.

28. Santucci B, Picardo M, Iavorone C et al., Contact dermatitis to *Alstroemeria*. *Contact Dermatitis* 1985; **12**:215–219.

29. Epstein E, *Primula* contact dermatitis: an easily overlooked diagnosis. *Cutis* 1990; **45**:411–416.

30. Garcia Ortiz JC, Terron M, Bellido J, Contact allergy to henna. *Int Arch Allergy Immunol* 1997; **114**:298–299.

31. Pasricha JS, Gupta R, Panjwani S, Contact dermatitis to henna (*Lawsonia*). *Contact Dermatitis* 1980; **6**:288–289.

32. Juckett G, Plant dermatitis. Possible culprits go far beyond poison ivy. *Postgrad Med* 1996; **100**:159–171.

33. Paulsen E, Occupational dermatitis in Danish gardeners and greenhouse workers. *Contact Dermatitis* 1998; **38**:14–19.

34. de Jong NW, Vermeulen AM, Gerth van Wijk R, de Groot H, Occupational allergy caused by flowers. *Allergy* 1998; **53**:204–209.

35. Mitchell JC, Maibach HI, Difficulties to investigate dermatitis from plants. *Dermatosen* 1996; **44**:29–33.

18. Photoallergic Contact Dermatitis

Ute Barta

Specific exogenous substances are activated by non-ionizing electromagnetic radiation, mostly UV A radiation, from sunlight or artificial UV sources, particularly sunbeds. They can cause photosensitization by different photochemical processes. The clinical result is a photosensitivity reaction. Substances that cause a photosensitivity reaction will be described in this chapter by the word "photosensitizers", more exactly they are termed "exogenous photosensitizers". These have to be distinguished from endogenous photosensitizers, which are produced in the body, for example in abnormal metabolism defects, such as porphyrias. Exogenous photosensitizers can enter the skin topically or systemically through parenteral application via the vascular system. Medications, UV-absorbing sunscreens, cosmetics, aftershaves, perfumes, nutrients and psoralen-containing plants can be exogenous photosensitizers.[1,2]

Two types of photosensitive reactions may occur, phototoxic or photoallergic. Phototoxic reactions are much more common than photoallergic reactions. The terms phototoxicity and photoallergy were introduced by Epstein in 1939[3] to differentiate several that occur after application of sulphanilamide plus exposure to sunlight. In both reaction types the photosensitizer acts as a chromophore, which absorbs UV energy and is converted into an energetically stimulated condition, the primary photoproduct. On the one hand, this photoproduct can work as a photoallergen, through conjugation with exogenous proteins, and cause a photoallergic reaction. On the other hand, it may react with photobiological substrates, directly or indirectly in combination with oxygen radicals. The subsequent biological condition is a phototoxic reaction.[4] Photosensitivity reactions have become increasingly common over recent decades, caused by changed life conditions and increasing amounts of photosensitizing chemicals in our environment. Pathological reactions of the photosensitized skin are usually caused by UV A radiation (320–400nm), and occasionally by visible light (400–790nm). Since windowpanes and thin textiles allow UV A and visible light to pass, photosensitivity reactions may even occur whilst driving a car or wearing thin clothes.[5]

Phototoxic reactions may occur following the first exposure to the photosensitizing chemical if the dose of chemical and appropriate radiation is high enough. Each person reacts differently. Acute phototoxic responses are usually characterized by clearly limited erythema on those parts of the body that are not protected by clothes, followed by hyperpigmentation and desquamation or peeling.

Photoallergic reactions are mostly delayed, T-cell mediated immunological reactions, which are classified as a type IV reaction according to Coombs and Gell.[6] Clinically, they usually appear as photoallergic contact dermatitis, more rarely as a photoallergic drug rash. The intensity depends on light exposure; therefore, they occur primarily in spring and summer.

Photoallergic contact dermatitis develops after repeated skin contact with photoallergens (photocontact allergens) plus exposure to sunlight or artificial UV sources. The clinical presentation is identical to any other type of allergic contact dermatitis (ACD). In the beginning, there is a clearly limited erythema, which may result in a severe vesiculobullous eruption within 24h, including itching papules and vesicles. When the process is chronic, scaling and lichenification can occur. Characteristically, the retroauricular area, the area under the chin (chin shadow) and areas that are covered by hair are not affected, in contrast to ACD and irritant contact dermatitis (ICD). The outer limits are less clear than in phototoxic reactions. The eruption may extend to unexposed parts of the skin (scattering) and even become generalized. However, the light-exposed areas are always the most affected.

The clinical presentation of photoallergic contact dermatitis is identical to that seen in ACD with oedema, perivascular lymphohistiocytic infiltrations in the cutis and spongiosis, as a chronic process with acanthosis and parakeratosis in the epidermis. Photoallergic drug eruptions after systemic application of the photoallergen are less common and less well understood than photoallergic contact dermatitis. The clinical eruptions range from lichenoid papules to eczematous changes with occasional lichenification on light-exposed skin.

In chronic cases, the systemic photoallergy is scarcely distinguishable from a photoallergic contact dermatitis. In general, removal of the photoallergen will eliminate the problem, and the eczematous skin eruptions heals after days, weeks or months, when the photoallergen is avoided. A small percentage of patients with photoallergic contact dermatitis develops a chronic dermatitis on light-exposed areas of the skin without apparent further contact with the photoallergen. The light sensitivity remains extremely high. Uncommon scattered reactions occur in covered skin areas. This is a persistent light reaction or chronic photosensitive dermatitis (Figure 18.1).[7] Clinically, the occurrence of persistent light reaction is the most important problem in photoallergy. This disease was described by Wilkinson in 1962.[8] It can persist over years and uncommonly change into actinic reticuloid, which is probably the final stage of chronic photosensitive dermatitis.[9] Persistent light reaction occurs mainly in middle-aged to elderly men, frequently in farmers, forestry workers or gardeners who have increased contact to plants. Skin eruptions may recede when the patient is no longer exposed to the formerly described radiation. The histology of actinic reticuloid is a spongiotic dermatitis with resemblance to T-cell lymphoma. The mechanism of persistent light reaction remains unclear.[10] In 1979, Hawk and

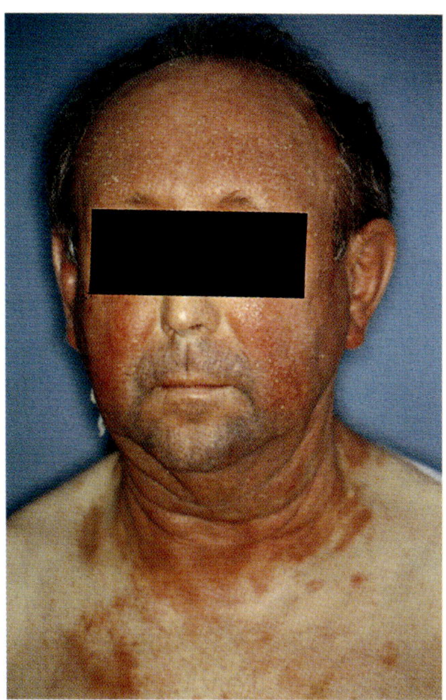

Figure 18.1: Persistent light reaction.

Magnus[11] suggested the term "chronic actinic dermatitis" for dermatitis on light-exposed skin as a result of chronic photosensitivity.[11]

Photoallergens

Frequent photocontact allergens are antibacterial and antifungal agents such as halogenated salicylanilides and related compounds, fragrances, and sunscreens containing chemical UV light filters. The most common causes of photoallergic contact dermatitis in Germany are UV light absorbing filters.[12,13] Light filters are contained in numerous cosmetics, creams, lipsticks and so on. They are not always declared. Because light filters are used for therapy of photodermatitis, the diagnosis of photoallergy is important. The most common systemic photoallergens include antibacterial sulphonamides, sulfonylurea antidiabetic medications, diuretic medications (especially hydrochlorothiazide), phenothiazines (in particular chlorpromazine), chinidin, chinin and certain antibiotics. Chronic systemic photoallergy is often found in older patients who take medicaments for hypertension, cardiac arrhythmia or diabetes mellitus and often stay outdoors.[14] Generally, substances that become known as photoallergens are eliminated from use. Therefore, photoallergic reactions can be observed frequently when substances are new to the market. There are geographical differences in the frequency of photoallergic reactions to special substances, because their use and the legislation varies in different countries.

Differential diagnosis

Differential diagnosis of photoallergic contact dermatitis includes any eruption, especially on light-exposed skin. The most important but often difficult differential diagnosis is airborne contact dermatitis due to the Compositae (Asteraceae), fragrances, etc., which characteristically but not always involves the so-called light shadow areas such as the eyelids, retroauricular area and the areas under the chin and behind the ears.[15] Other differential diagnoses are phototoxic reactions, eczema of other origin, and especially the eczematous type of polymorphous light reactions.

Diagnosis

If the history and clinical presentation indicate a photoallergic dermatitis, this diagnosis should be proved. The most reliable diagnostic tool is the photopatch test, which identifies the photosensitizers. It is also advisable if chronic actinic dermatitis is suspected. The photopatch test is a special form of the patch test.[16] The recommended test substances depend on region-specific photoallergens and must be adapted to the current conditions and knowledge.

Photopatch testing was introduced by Schultz et al.[17] and Epstein and Rowe.[18] Nowadays, the test has a firm place in dermatologic diagnostics. It was not standardized until the 1980s. The first attempt to standardize the test was initiated by the Scandinavian Photodermatitis Group in 1982.[19,20] In 1984, 45 dermatological centres in Germany, Austria and Switzerland founded the Photopatch Test Group (Arbeitsgemeinschaft Photopatch-Test, DAPT), which elaborated a new standardized test procedure, as described here.[21–24] In Table 18.1, this test procedure is shown. The potential photoallergens are applied on the back of the patient in double test series, using small aluminium patches (Finn-Chambers Scanpor, Hermal, Reinbek bei Hamburg). One set of patches is irradiated with 10J/cm^2 UV A light 24h after application. Another set of patches serves as a non-irradiated dark test sample to exclude a non-photosensitive contact dermatitis. It is advisable to start with UV A light-testing minimal erythema dose (MED). The irradiation has to be executed using a suberythematous UV A dose. The irradiation dose of 10J/cm^2 is relatively high, and probably favours the development of phototoxic reactions; most other study groups preferred doses of 3–5J/cm^2.[19] Readings are performed immediately

Table 18.1 Photopatch test procedure

Test localization	Back
Duration of application	24h
UV dose	10J/cm^2 UV A, or lower if MED for UV A $<$10J/cm^2
Readings	Immediately and 24, 48 and 72h later
Controls	Non-irradiated patch test

Table 18.2 Evaluation of the photopatch test

0 = No reaction
1 = Erythema
2 = Erythema and dermal infiltrate
3 = Erythema and papulovesicles
4 = Erythema, bullae, erosions

before and after the irradiation as well as on successive days, up to 72h later, sometimes with additional readings 1–2 weeks later. The test reactions are evaluated by morphological criteria, not by intensity (Table 18.2). An erythema is an already relevant reaction.[24] This differs from the recommendations of the International Contact Dermatitis Group.

The following reaction types are possible:[24]

- **Photoallergic reaction:** erythema, infiltration, possible papulovesicles only on the irradiated area; crescendo pattern; no reaction on non-irradiated areas, or considerable difference between irradiated and non-irradiated areas
- **Allergic reaction:** infiltration, possible papulovesicles; equal reactions on both sides; crescendo pattern
- **Light-increased allergic reaction:** reaction on the irradiated site is more intensive and/or persistent for longer than on the non irradiated site; both contact and photocontact allergy can exist at the same time (turn over point 1)
- **Phototoxic reaction:** erythema and oedema only on the irradiated site; decrescendo pattern
- **Toxic reaction:** erythema and oedema of the same intensity on both irradiated on non-irradiated sites, independent of irradiation

The relevance of test reactions can only be assessed in the context of profound knowledge of case history and presentation. The most frequent problem is how to differentiate between a phototoxic and a photoallergic reaction. In case of

Table 18.3 Standard photoallergens

Photoallergen	*Concentration (% pet)*
Tetrachlorosalicylanilide	0.1
Bromochlorosalicylanilide	1.0
Hexachlorophene	1.0
Bithionol	1.0
Sulphanilamide	5.0
Promethazine hydrochloride	0.1
Quinidine sulphate	1.0
Musk ambrette	5.0
Perfume mix	8.0
4-Aminobenzoic acid	10.0
2-Ethylhexyl-4-dimethylaminobenzoate	10.0
4-tert-Butyl-4'-methoxy-dibenzoylmethane	10.0
Isoamyl-4-methoxycinnamate	10.0
2-Ethylhexyl-4-methoxycinnamate	10.0
3-(4-Methylbenzylidene)-camphor	10.0
2-Phenylbenzimidazol-5-sulphonic acid	10.0
Benzophenone-3 (Oxybenzone)	10.0
Benzophenone-4 (Sulisobenzon)	10.0
Additional test substances	
Tribromsalicylanilide	1.0
Chlorpromazine hydrochloride	0.1
Thiourea	0.1
Olaquindox	1.0

doubt, it is possible to do a serial dilution series of the suspected photoallergen and also to vary the dose of irradiation. A positive reaction at a very low concentration and/or very low light dose is typical of photoallergy.[15] But it is known that most photosensitizers are capable of inducing both reactions, photoallergic and phototoxic. Table 18.3 gives the standard photoallergens, which were suggested by the Photopatch Test Group.[25] This standard series comprises the substances that have most frequently been identified as photoallergens, in relevant concentrations. They are commercially distributed by Hermal (Germany) and may be used as a matter of routine if photoallergy is suspected. Chemotechnique (Sweden) offers a sunscreen series that can also be used (see Chapter 21).

Topical or sytemic drugs used by the patient which are potential photosensitizers should also be tested. The test area must be clinically healthy. Until 3 weeks before the photopatch test, topical therapy with corticosteroids and intensive sun exposure should be avoided. Any systemic therapy with corticosteroids and antihistamines should be finished 1 week before photopatch testing. Photopatch testing is not suitable for recognition of systemic photosensitizers, often causing false-negative testing results; possible causes are insufficient penetration through the horn barrier of the skin and the fact that metabolites of the medication are the real photosensitizers, so that only a systemic photo-provocation test may clarify the connection between the drug and light. After re-exposure to the drug in question graduated irradiation with UV A and UV B is carried out.

A total-body light provocation test is also possible, but has a higher risk.[26,27] Histological examination of both the primary skin change and the testing reaction improves the exactness of diagnosis. If photosensitivity is suspected but the photopatch test is negative, a modified photopatch test after tape stripping, or a scratch, prick or intradermal test can be done, because systemic provocation can be dangerous and more lasting persistent light sensitivity can follow.[28] In light-exposed intradermal testing, the substance in question is intradermally injected in suitable dilution and in tolerable vehicles and 15 min later irradiated with a UV A dose lower than the MED. Readings are performed immediately before and after the irradiation as well as on successive days up to 72h. To differentiate between phototoxic and photoallergic reactions it is necessary to have non-irradiated test samples as well as tests on test patients. The following procedure is advisable if a systemic exogenous photoallergy is suspected:[28]

1. UV light testing with UV A and UV B (MED-determination) under application of potential photosensitizer or a short time after its discontinuation, as well as some weeks later
2. Photopatch testing
3. Modified patch testing (patch test on tape-stripped skin, on scratch or prick)
4. Irradiated intradermal testing
5. Systemic photoprovocation

Therapy

The therapy of acute photocontact dermatitis is similar to that of ACD. This includes the use of topical "cool cloths", wet dressings, soothing shake lotions, topical corticosteroids. Systemic antihistamines as well as systemic corticosteroids may by indicated. Therapy of chronic photosensitive dermatitis, especially of actinic reticuloid is difficult. Psoralen photochemotherapy, the combination of the photoactive drug psoralen (P), with long-wave UV light (UV A), has a good effect.[29] Combination with immunosuppressive drugs may be necessary. The most important measure is avoidance of the photosensitizer, if it is known.

It is essential to avoid sun. Light protection has to be maintained as long as the light sensitivity exists. The best measure is the light protection by suitable textiles as well as physical light protection, because it eliminates the risk of photoallergy. For patients with severe actinic reticuloid there are UV-permeable sun protection foils in the form of blinds or to be stuck on windowpanes.

References

1. Schauder S, Ippen H, Photosensitivität. In: Fuchs E, Schulz KH, eds. *Manuale allergologicum* München-Deisenhofen: Dustri-Verlag; 1988:1–30.
2. Johnson BE, Drug and chemical photosenzitisation. In: Marks R, Plewig G, eds. *The environmental threat to the skin*. London: Dunitz; 1992:57–65.
3. Epstein S, Photoallergy and primary phototoxicity to sulfanilamide. *J Invest Dermatol* 1939; **2**:43–51.
4. Goerz G, Merk HF, Hölzle E, Photoallergy. In: Krutmann J, Elmets CA, eds. 1995:176–186.
5. Lischka G, Jung EG, *Lichtkrankheiten der Haut*. Erlangen: Perimed Verlag; 1982:••–••.
6. Coombs RRA, Gell PGH, Classification of allergic reactions responsible for clinical hypersensitivity and disease. In: Gell PGH, Coombs RRA, Lachmann PJ, eds. *Clinical aspects of immunology*. Oxford: Blackwell Scientific Publications; 1975:761.
7. Frain-Bell W, Lakshmipathi T, Rogers J, Willock J, The syndrome of chronic photosensitivity dermatitis and actinic reticuloid. *Br J Dermatol* 1974; **91**:617–634.
8. Wilkinson DS, Patch test reactions to certain halogenated salicylanilides. *Br J Dermatol* 1962; **74**:302–306.
9. Wolf C, Hönigsmann H, Persistierende Lichtreaktion-aktinisches Retikuloid als Syndrom der chronisch aktinischen Dermatitis. *Hautarzt* 1988; **39**:635–641.
10. Ive FA, Magnus IA, Warin RP,Wilson Jones E, Actinic reticuloid, a chronic dermatosis associated with severe photosensitivity and the histological resemblance to lymphoma. *Br J Dermatol* 1969; **81**:469–485.
11. Hawk JLM, Magnus IA, Chronic actinic dermatitis – an idiopathic photosensitivity syndrome including actinic reticuloid and photosensitive eczema. *Br J Dermatol* 1979; **101 (suppl 17)**:24.
12. Schauder S, Basiswissen Photoallergie. *Allergololgie* 1996; **19**:556–559.
13. Schauder S, Schrader H, Ippen H, *Göttinger Liste 1996 – Sonnenschutzkosmetik in Deutschland*. Berlin: Blackwell; 1996:51–55.

14. Schauder S, Chronische photoallergische Dermatosen. *Dermatol Monatsschr* 1992; **178**:245–254.

15. White IR, Photoallergens and photosensitivity: current problems. In: Marks R, Plewig G, eds. *The environmental threat to the skin*. London: Dunitz; 1992:51–55.

16. Hölzle E, Rowold J, Peter S, Plewig G, Die belichtete Epikutantestung. *Allergologie* 1989; **12**:13–20.

17. Schultz KH, Wiskemann K, Wolf K, Klinische und experimentelle Untersuchungen über die photodynamische Wirksamkeit von Phenothiazinderivaten, insbesondere Megaphen. *Arch Klin Exp Dermatol* 1956; **202**:285–298.

18. Epstein S, Rowe RJ, Photoallergy and photocross-sensitivity to phenergan. *J Invest Dermatol* 1957; **29**:319–326.

19. Jansen CT, Wennersten G, Tystedt I et al., The Scandinavian standard photopatch test procedure. *Contact Dermatitis* 1982; **8**:155–158.

20. Thune A, Jansen C, Wennersten G et al., The Scandinavian multicenter photopatch test study 1980–1985: final report. *Photodermatology* 1988; **5**:261–269.

21. Lehmann P, Die Deutschsprachige Arbeitsgemeinschaft Photopatch-Test (DAPT). *Hautarzt* 1990; **41**:295–297.

22. Hölzle E und die Mitglieder der Deutschsprachigen Arbeitsgemeinschaft Photopatch-Test, Photopatch-Test: Ergebnisse der multizentrischen Studie. *Akt Dermatol* 1991; **17**:117–123.

23. Hölzle E, Meumann N, Hausen B et al., Photopatch testing: the 5-year experience of the German, Austrian and Swiss photopatch test group. *J Am Acad Dermatol* 1991; **25**:59–68.

24. Neumann N, Hölzle E, Lehmann P et al., Pattern analysis of photopatch test reactions. *Photodermatol Photoimmunol Photomed* 1994; **10**:65–73.

25. Rünger TM, Lehmann P, Neumann NJ et al., Empfehlungen einer Photopatch-Test Standardreihe durch die deutschsprachige Arbeitsgruppe “Photopatch-Test”. *Hautarzt* 1995; **46**:240–243.

26. Hölzle E, Plewig G, Lehmann P, Photodermatosis – diagnostic procedures and their interpretation. *Photodermatology* 1986; **4**:109–114.

27. Lehmann P, Hölzle E, von Kries R et al., Lichtdiagnostische Verfahren bei Patienten mit Verdacht auf Photodermatosen. *Zentralbl Haut* 1986; **152**:667–682.

28. Schauder S, Der modifizierte intradermale Test im Vergleich zu anderen Verfahren zum Nachweis von phototoxischen und photoallergischen Arzneireaktionen. *Z Hautkr* 1990; **65**:247–255.

29. Galosi A, Hölzle E, Plewig G, Braun-Falco O, PUVA-Therapie bei persistierender Lichtreaktion. *Hautarzt* 1982; **33**:657–661.

19. Miscellaneous Contact Allergens

Annett Looks and Matthias Gebhardt

This chapter covers a heterogeneous group of miscellaneous substances that each need to be mentioned but does not justify its own chapter. The allergens described here have allergenic importance in occupations, hobbies, sports, leisure time, the household and medicine. They include tars and balms, plastics, especially epoxy resins and acrylates, glues and adhesives, photochemicals and azo dyes.

Tars and balsams

Tars (wood tar and coal tar) and balsams are naturally occurring materials that are prevalent both at work and in leisure-time activities. In addition, although known for their potential health risks, coal-tar derivates are still used to treat psoriasis and other dermatoses. Various ointments for leg ulcers, plasters, suppositories and cosmetics may contain balsamic compounds such as balsam of Peru and balsam of Tolu, or at least the allergenic ingredients of these, e.g. cinnamic aldehyde, cinnamic acid and benzoic acid.

Allergic contact dermatitis (ACD) from coal tar, though rare, has been reported, while irritant reactions are quite common. Tar irritation is often a pustular or follicular rash. Rudzki and Grzywa[1] and Conde-Salazar et al.[2] have described true occupational ACD which occurred after long-standing skin contact at work. Sensitization by treatment of chronic inflammatory skin disorders like psoriasis or eczema is not unlikely after years of treatment[3] but has even been seen after a short period.[4] Cross sensitization between various tars and balsams is common, on the basis of their shared ingredients. Roesyanto et al.[5] found concomitant reactions of wood and coal tars in 18.5%, wood tars and fragrance mix in 43%, and wood tars and balsam of Peru in 31% of a population of 1883 test patients for ACD. These results emphasize the indicator role of fragrance mix or any tar for the entire chemical group of tars and balsams. Tar allergy may also be caused by perfume intolerance. Impurities in the raw material of tar test substances, tar's crossreactivity with well-characterized substances and, not least, debate on the carcinogenicity of tars has lead to diminishing role for tar patch tests in the last few years.

A commercially available test series, "tars and balsams", is shown in Table 19.1. The standard screening patch test series of any provider includes balsam

Table 19.1 The test series 'tars and balsams'

Substances	*Test concentration (%)*
Coal tar	3
Birch wood tar	3
Beech wood tar	3
Juniper wood tar	3
Pine wood tar	3
Styrax	2
Pine balsam	20
Spruce balsam	20
Balsam of Tolu	20
Larch terpentine	20

of Peru as a common indicator of fragrance sensitivity. Despite their controversial role, tar patch tests should be performed in patients suspected of having contact allergy to coal tar in order to exclude irritant contact dermatitis (ICD) or photosensitization. If irritation cannot be ruled out definitely in a positive test reaction to coal tar, it is wise to do a dilution series down to a coal tar concentration of 0.1%.

Plastics

Plastics (synthetic resins) consist of polymers that are long chains of molecules linked together in a polymerization process. In this process, a wide range of chemicals may be added, among them curing agents, stabilizers, plasticizers, catalysts, accelerators and antioxidants. Several of these chemicals may be irritants or sensitizers themselves. As is the case for many other contact allergens, plastics may cause dermatitis, both ACD and ICD. Skin hazards are almost exclusively caused by uncured plastics, not the final products. The most important sources of contact allergy due to plastics are:

- Epoxy resin
- Formaldehyde resin
- Polyurethane
- (Meth)acrylates

Many of the allergenic plastics are used as glues. Test series therefore usually combine glues, adhesives and plastics in the same test tray.

Table 19.2 Plastic additives with sensitizing capacity: test recommendations

Phthalates
Maleates
Cobalt naphthenate
Benzoyl peroxide
Dimethylaniline
Toluene sulphonic acid
Paraphenylendiamine derivates
Mercaptobenzothiazole
Phenols
Epoxy resins, hardeners

Polyester plastics are common irritants but seldom allergens. Table 19.2 shows plastic additives which should be considered when composing test trays for plastic-induced contact dermatitis.

As mentioned above, the solid, cured or fully polymerized synthetic resin rarely causes dermatitis. In the manufacture of plastics, contact with uncured resins, catalysts and additives is however unavoidable. Therefore, contact dermatitis to plastics is mainly of occupational or hobby origin. Currently, epoxy and acrylic resins are among the most important sources of occupational contact dermatitis. Occupational relevance is found in construction workers, dental personnel, car manufacturers, the plastic industry, etc. In addition to simple contact dermatitis induced by skin contact with uncured plastics, contact urticaria and allergic or irritant airborne contact dermatitis caused by volatile compounds have been described.[6]

In the following, we would like to give emphasis to some examples relevant in a dermatologist's ordinary practice.

Epoxy resin

First we will look at epoxy resin contact reactions. Epoxy resins occur mostly in the construction, chemical (paints and adhesives), car, ship, aeroplane, sports equipment and optical industries, and in the manufacture of electrical equipment for enclosing transformers, condensers, etc. As specific examples, epoxy resin has been proven to be a potential allergen in the working process in a ski-stick factory;[7] Holness and Nethercott[8] reported occupational contact dermatitis due to epoxy resin in a fibreglass binder. These examples illustrate the possibility of encountering epoxy resin use in industrial fields in which heavy duty equipment is produced. An almost classic field of epoxy resin is construction work,[9] e.g. flooring,[10] marble[11] and chipboard work.[12]

There are frequent reports of non-occupational cases of epoxy resin sensitivity, too. Contact dermatitis due to epoxy resin in knee patch adhesive in a boy's jeans,[13] in a bowlsgrip,[14] and in textile labels[15] have been published, just to give a few examples of its increasing use in everyday products.

Epoxy resins are often two-component systems. They are not sensitizing when fully cured but frequently contain an amount of remaining monomer which is sufficient to boost a pre-existing sensitization. Chemically, most epoxy resin is based on bisphenol A and epichlorhydrin. Hardeners of the amine or acid anhydride type are added as cross-linkers into the resin. In contrast with the consumer, it is the people engaged in working processes involving epoxy resins who are much more affected by allergies.

We recommend that patch tests with epoxy chemicals are limited to the standardized test series because of the danger of active sensitization. Once proven, epoxy resins should not be re-tested, in our opinion. When testing epoxy-exposed people, one should never forget to include chemical additives such as the broad range of hardeners.

Acrylates

Acrylates are considered the fourth most common cause of contact sensitization due to resin. They have extensive applications in various products such as paints, oil additives, textiles, lenses, windows, cosmetics, and in medicine and dentistry. Their excellent properties such as strong sticking power (even to metals, ceramics, glass and other building materials), fast curing and easy handling make them a first choice for industrial adhesives. Stickers, tapes and office material may also be based on acrylic adhesives. Unpolymerized monomers of acrylic compounds are known to be responsible for contact allergy. There is a controversy about the so-called rest monomer in cured acrylates and its role in the initiation and elicitation of contact allergy. Accelerators, inhibitors and catalysts, which are added to the acrylates, can also sensitize. Other macromolecular substances may be included with acrylates, such as epoxy resins to form epoxy acrylates.

It may be difficult to find suitable personal protective equipment for sensitized people because most acrylates do easily penetrate gloves. In addition to allergy, irritation contributes to the hazardous health effects of acrylates.

Patch testing with plastics

Epoxy resin is part of the standard series; in addition there are special series for synthetic resins/adhesives and acrylates. Patch testing can produce active sensitization to patch test allergens, especially in testing acrylics[16] and epoxy resins.[17] The concentration of patch test substances should be as low as possible though high enough to confirm contact allergy, especially in patch testing with unknown chemicals such as the patient's own substances.[18] Testing the patient's own products is not recommended in routine practice. Recently, it has been found that the special series reveal the cause of ACD less frequently than the standard series.[19] Once epoxy sensitization has been confirmed, to avoid strong booster reactions one should not re-test the individual.

A test screening with several acrylates should be done when acrylate allergy is suspected. Chemotechnique has the most diverse patch test tray for methacrylates; however, the other companies also provide a suitable screening composition. As early as 1975 Jordan[20] recommended that methyl methacrylate alone is not a good screening for acrylate allergy.

Adhesives

Many modern adhesives are two-component systems based on polymerization of synthetic macromolecular substances. Synthetic organic adhesives are grouped on the basis of their chemical structure, according to White[21] (Table 19.3).

Para-tertiary butylphenol formaldehyde resin (PTBP-FR) is a well-known allergen with particular use as a neoprene-based leather glue. Therefore it has occupational relevance for shoemakers. An Italian survey revealed PTBP-FR containing neoprene adhesives to be the major allergen in a shoe factory.[22] PTBP-FR-based glues have also been reported for their use in car manufacture.[23] Non-occupational relevance is found in foot dermatitis elicited by shoes, wrist dermatitis by watch straps and other leather articles.[24] For patch test purposes, PTBP-FR is available 1% pet.

Ureaformaldehyde resin and **melamine formaldehyde resin** are used as glues in the wood industries to make furniture press plates. Construction

Table 19.3 Synthetic organic adhesives

Acrylates
Vinyl resins
Cellulose derivates
Polyester derivates
Phenol resin adhesives
Amino formaldehyde polymers
Epoxy resins
Polyimide and polyamide adhesives
Polyurethanes
Elastomeric adhesives

workers are exposed to formaldehyde resins in modern building materials as well. Textile finishes are another use of these formaldhehyde resins.

Toluenesulphonamide formaldehyde resin (TS-FR) is a very common ingredient of nail lacquers and hardeners. It may be an occupational allergen for cosmetic artists and beauticians and, of course, an allergen for the consumer. Typically, TS-FR allergy involves the eyelids, lateral aspects of the neck and more rarely the most exposed periungual area. Because traces of the allergen are easily transferred to the eyelids, it has been included in the topical eye preparation series of several test allergen providers.

Glues based on **acrylates** are widely used as contact adhesives for metal, glass, rubber, plastics and textiles, as well as for biological materials such as binding tissues and sealing wounds in surgery.[25] In sticking something to glass, ceramics or metal surfaces, 2-hydroxy ethyl methacrylate (2-HEMA), 2-hydroxy propyl methacrylate (2-HPMA) and (tri)ethylene glycol dimethacrylate (TEGDMA or EGDMA) are common ingredients of industrial adhesives.[26] Cyanoacrylates are among the most common ingredients of acrylate "super glues" or "crazy glues". Eyelid eczema, nummular eczema on the hands and periungual dermatitis are typical features of ACD caused by cyanoacrylate glue used to fix artificial nails. Ethyl cyanoacrylate and methyl methacrylate have been seen as allergens in these patients.[27,28]

Colophony rosin, a naturally occurring rosin from trees, is another natural base of glues and adhesives. Abietic acid, also available as test allergen, and its oxidative derivatives are the causative allergens.[29] It is high ranking in target lists of contact allergens because of widespread exposure, ranging from occupational use in electronics, wood, paper, paint and the cosmetics industries through household contact and on to natural exposure.[30] Medical use of rosin derivatives on tapes, bandages, surgical and dental dressings, wart paints and hydrocolloid dressings has been reported.[31,32] Most patients with a sensitization to colophony report intolerance of brown-coloured tapes.

Photochemicals

Colour development photochemicals chemically related to paraphenylenediamine are well-known sensitizers (Table 19.4). Crossreactivity between the colour film developers has been reported.[33]

Sensitization to several developers may result in eczema or, as a special pattern of contact allergy, to lichenoid dermatitis mainly of the hands, arms and face. The exposure is either direct or airborne.[34,35] As early as 1959 Canizares described a systemic contact dermatitis due to the inhalation of colour film developers.[36] Because of their limited use, only a few people are exposed to these chemicals at work or in leisure time.[37] Nowadays, more and more film

Table 19.4 Colour developer screening substances

Commercial name	*Chemical name*
CD 2	*N,N*-Diethyl-*p*-phenylene diamine hydrochlorid
CD 3	4-(*N*-Ethyl-*N*-2-methanesulphonylaminoethyl)-2-methyl-*p*-phenylenediamine sesquisulphate monohydrate
CD 4	4-(*N*-Ethyl-*N*-2-hydroxyethyl)-2-methylphenylenediamine sulphate

developing is automated with the use of encapsulated film processors. So these allergens are less important today than they were in past years.

Colour development agents are unstable in water solutions. Therefore patch testing should be done with petrolatum preparations.[38] Long-standing patch test reactions are not uncommon and lichenoid reactions may occur. Photographic test series are commercially available.

Azo dyes

Another well-characterized group of chemicals, the azo-dyes, have less and less use, currently. There are health concerns, which make them less suitable for consumer products. However, until recently, these colouring chemicals were frequently used in textiles and clothing (Figures 19.1 and 19.2), cosmetics (e.g. lipsticks), foods and the paper industry. Moreover, azo compounds may be contained in hair dye, coloured furs and leather, printer's ink, photographic products, X-ray fluids and lithographs.[39]

Sensitization to azo dyes may be due to the azo dye itself or to its degradation products. Concomitant reaction with different azo dyes could either be based on true cross sensitization or on separate sensitization.[40] Impurities in the raw materials, e.g. contamination of one dye by another, presumably may account for more cross reactions. Disperse dyes of the azo type have been reported to crossreact with *para*-amino compounds.[41]

The hands, neck, face, axillae, lower and upper limbs, and trunk are the most frequently involved skin sites in patients allergic to azo dyes, depending on the contact area. The most important allergens in the the azo dyes used in textiles are disperse yellow 3, disperse orange 3 and disperse red 1, which are used in stocking and tights. These dyes have a low sensitizing potency in contrast to the strong sensitizers disperse blue 106 and 124, which are used in blouses and trousers. Several azo dyes are contaminated by others, which explains the high rate of concomitant reactions.

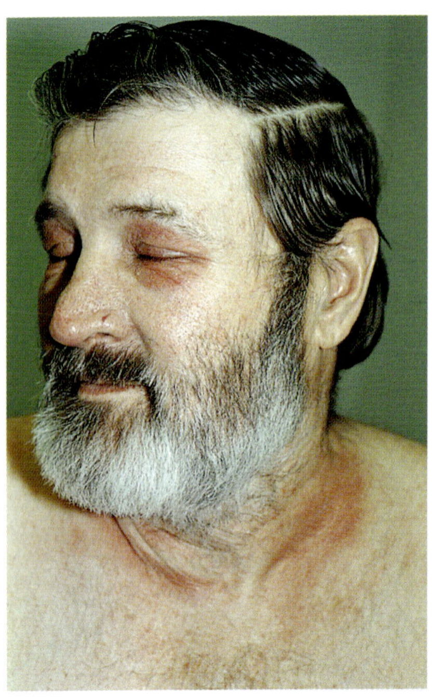

Figure 19.1: Allergic contact dermatitis to textile dye.

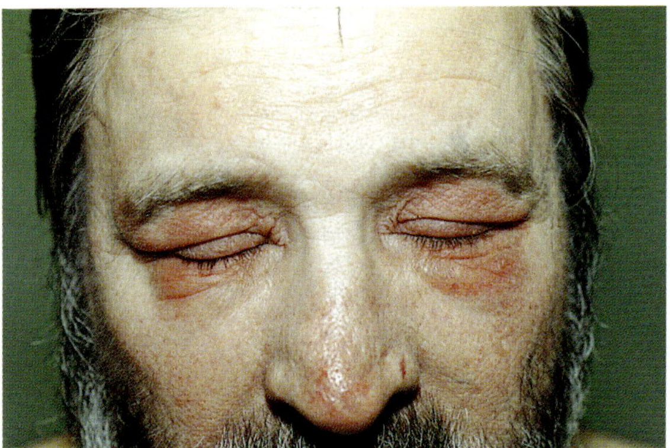

Figure 19.2: Allergic contact dermatitis to textile dye.

Azo dyes may also be important in hairdresser's hand dermatitis. Disperse orange 3 used in hair dyes is the allergen most commonly responsible.

Urticaria, angioneurotic oedema and contact urticaria caused by azo dyes as additives in food[42] and contact dermatitis to azo–naphthol dyes contained in sunscreens[43] are less common. For testing procedure see Chapter 13. Hermal offers an organic dye series and textile dye series. The controversial role of paraphenylenediamine as an indicator allergen in the standard series is discussed in the literature.[44]

References

1. Rudzki E, Grzywa Z, Occupational dermatitis partly elicited by coal tar. *Contact Dermatitis* 1977; **3**:54.

2. Conde-Salazar L, Guimaraens D, Romero LV, Gozalez MA, Occupational coal tar dermatitis. *Contact Dermatitis* 1987; **16**:231.

3. Riboldi A, Pigatto PD, Innocenti M et al., Contact dermatitis to coal tar in psoriasis. *Contact Dermatitis* 1990; **14**:187–188.

4. Cusano F, Capozzi M, Errico G, Allergic contact dermatitis from coal tar. *Contact Dermatitis* 1992; **27**:51–52.

5. Roesyanto ID, van den Akker TW, van Jost TW, Wood tars allergy, cross-sensitization and coal tar. *Contact Dermatitis* 1990; **22**:95–98.

6. Tosti A, Guerra L, Vincenzi C, Peluso AM, Occupational skin hazards from synthetic plastics. *Toxicol Ind Health* 1993; **9**:493–502.

7. Suhonen R, Epoxy dermatitis in a ski-stick factory. *Contact Dermatitis* 1983, **9**:131–133.

8. Holness DL, Nethercott JR, Occupational contact dermatitis due to epoxy resin in a fiberglass binder. *J Occup Med* 1989; **31**:87–89.

9. Conde-Salazar L, Guimaraens D, Villegas C et al., Occupational allergic contact dermatitis in construction workers. *Contact Dermatitis* 1995; **44**:226–230.

10. Conde-Salazar L, Gonzales de Domingo MA, Guimaraens D, Sensitization to epoxy resins systems in special flooring workers. *Contact Dermatitis* 1994; **31**:157–160.

11. Angelini G, Rigano L, Foti C et al., Occupational sensitization to epoxy resin and reactive diluents in marble workers. *Contact Dermatitis* 1996; **35**:11–16.

12. Goulden V, Wilkinson SM, Occupational allergic contact dermatitis from epoxy resin on chipboard. *Contact Dermatitis* 1996; **35**:262–263.

13. Taylor JS, Bergfeld WF, Guin JD, Contact dermatitis to knee patch adhesive in boy's jeans. A nonoccupational cause of epoxy resin sensitivity. *Cleve Clin Q* 1983; **50**:123–127.

14. Blair C, The dermatological hazards of bowling. Contact dermatitis to resin in a bowlsgrip. *Contact Dermatitis* 1982; **8**:138–139.

15. Fregert S, Orsmark K, Allergic contact dermatitis due to epoxy resin in textile labels. *Contact Dermatitis* 1984; **11**:131–132.

16. Kanerva, L, Estlander T, Jolanki R, Active sensitization caused by 2-hydroxyethyl methacrylate, 2-hydroxypropyl methacrylate, ethylenglycol dimethacrylate and *N,N*-dimethylaminoethyl methacrylate. *J Eur Acad Derm Venereol* 1992; **1**:165–169.

17. Jolanki R, Occupational skin diseases from epoxy compounds. Epoxy resin compounds, epoxy acrylates and 2,3-epoxypropyl trimethyl ammonium chloride. *Acta Derm Venereol* 1991; **suppl 159**:24.

18. Jolanki R, Tarvainen K, Tatar T et al., Occupational dermatoses from exposure to epoxy resin compounds in ski factory. *Contact Dermatitis* 1996; **34**:390–396.

19. Tarvainen K, Analysis of patients with allergic patch test reactions to a plastics and glues series. *Contact Dermatitis* 1995; **32**:346–351.

20. Jordan WP, Cross-sensitization patterns in acrylate allergies. *Contact Dermatitis* 1975; **1**:13–15.

21. White IR, Adhesives. In: Adams RM, ed. *Occupational skin disease*, 2nd edn. Philadelphia: WB Saunders; 1990:395–407.

22. Manusco G, Reggiani M, Berdondini RM, Occupational dermatitis in shoemakers. *Contact Dermatitis* 1996; **34**:17–22.

23. Schubert H, Agatha G, Zur Allergennatur der *para*-tert. Butylphenolformaldehydharze. *Dermatosen* 1979; **27**:49–52.

24. Freeman S, Shoe dermatitis. *Contact Dermatitis* 1997; **36**:247–251.

25. Bruze M, Björkner B, Lepoittevin JP, Occupational allergic contact dermatitis from ethyl cyanoacrylate. *Contact Dermatitis* 1995; **32**:156–159.

26. Kanerva L, Jolanki R, Leino T, Estlander T, Occupational allergic contact dermatitis from 2-hydroxyethyl methacrylate and ethylene glycol dimethacrylate in a modified acrylic structural adhesive. *Contact Dermatitis* 1995; **33**:84–89.

27. Belsito DV, Contact dermatitis to ethyl-cyanoacrylate-containing glue. *Contact Dermatitis* 1987; **17**:234–236.

28. Guin JD, Baas K, Nelson-Adesokan P, Contact sensitization to cyanoacrylate adhesive as a cause of severe onychodystrophy. *Int J Dermatol* 1998; **37**:31–36.

29. Guin JD, Colophony (Rosin). In: Guin JD, ed. *Practical contact dermatitis*. New York: McGraw-Hill Inc; 1995:115–124.

30. Sadhra S, Foulds IS, Gray CN et al., Colophony uses, health effects, airborne measurement and analysis. *Ann Occup Hyg* 1994; **38**:385–396.

31. Lachapelle JM, Leroy B, Allergic contact dermatitis to colophony included in the formulation of flexible collodion BP, the vehicle of a salicylic and lactic acid wart paint. *Dermatol Clin* 1990; **8**:143–146.

32. Sasseville D, Tennstedt D, Lachapelle JM, Allergic contact dermatitis from hydrocolloid dressings. *Am J Contact Dermatitis* 1997; **8**:236–238.

33. Liden C, Boman A, Contact allergy to colour developing agents in the guinea pig. *Contact Dermatitis* 1988; **19**:290–295.

34. Galindo PA, Garcia R, Gariindo JA et al., Allergic contact dermatitis from colour developers: absence of cross-sensitivity to *para*-amino compounds. *Contact Dermatitis* 1994; **30**:301.

35. Brancaccio RR, Cockerell CJ, Belsito D, Ostreicher R, Allergic contact dermatitis from color film developers: clinical and histologic features. *J Am Acad Dermatol* 1993; **28**:827–830.

36. Canizares O, Lichen planus-like erution caused by color developer. *Arch Dermatol* 1959; **80**:81–86.

37. Hansson C, Ahlfors S, Bergendorff O, Concomitant contact dermatitis due to textile dyes and to colour film developers can be explained by the formation of the same hapten. *Contact Dermatitis* 1997; **37**:27–31.

38. Sollenberg J, Liden C, Hansen L, Arvidson A, Contact allergy to colour developing agents. Analysis of test preparations, bulk chemicals and tank solutions by high-performance liquid chromatography. *Derm Beruf Umwelt* 1989; **37**:47–52.

39. Hatch KL, Maibach HI, Textile dye dermatitis. *J Am Acad Dermatol* 1995; **32**:631–639.

40. Seidenari S, Mantovani L, Manzini BM, Pignatti M, Cross-sensitizations between azo-dyes and *para*-amino compounds. *Contact Dermatitis* 1997; **36**:91–96.

41. Nakagawa M, Kawai K, Kawai K, Mutilple azo dye sensitization mainly due to group sensitization to azo dyes. *Contact Dermatitis* 1996; **34**:6–11.

42. Hannuksela M, Haathela T, Hypersensitivity reactions to food additives. *Allergy* 1987; **42**:561–575.

43. Thune P, Contact and photocontact allergy to sunscreens. *Photodermatol* 1984; **1**:5–9.

44. Thierbach MA, Geursen-Reitsma AM, van Jost T, Sensitization to azo dyes. Negative patch tests to yellow and red azo dyes in printed paper. *Contact Dermatitis* 1992; **27**:22–26.

20. Treatment Options in Recalcitrant Contact Dermatitis

Undine Berndt

Whilst acute contact dermatitis (ACD) can be treated successfully, the persistent case of eczema raises the greatest problems in management. Because the hands are often affected, many patients have to change their occupation or sometimes even retire resulting in individual problems and considerable costs to society. Figures 20.1 to 20.3 show examples of chronic contact dermatitis.

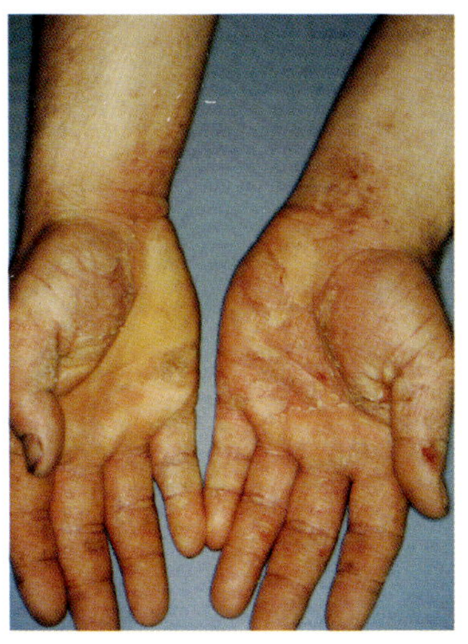

Figure 20.1: Chronic occupational hand dermatitis in a baker.

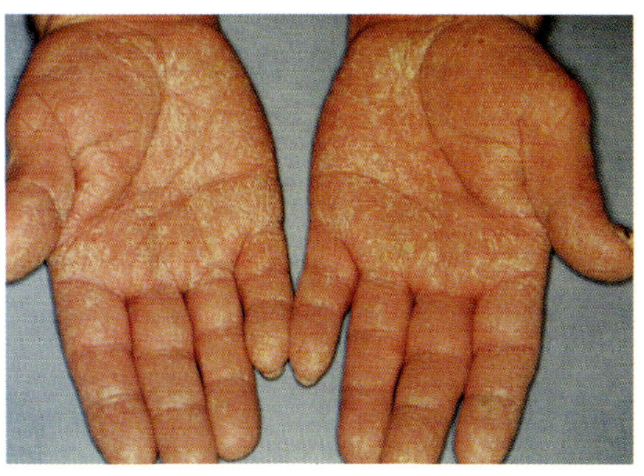

Figure 20.2: Chronic hyperkeratotic hand dermatitis due to chromate sensitization.

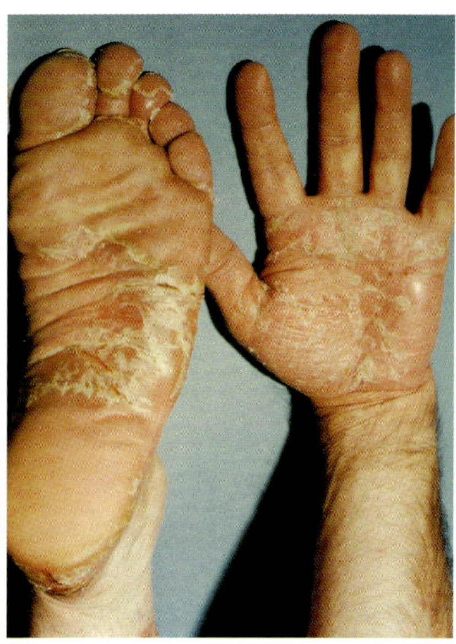

Figure 20.3: Chronic dermatitis of hands and feet in a patient with an atopic background.

If eczema shows an unusually recalcitrant course the correctness of the diagnosis should be questioned. Several common itchy skin conditions, such as psoriasis or fungal infection, may resemble eczematous symptoms.[1] Furthermore, the cause of the ongoing dermatitis has to be evaluated in great detail, including possible irritants or sensitizers as well as constitutional and modifying environmental co-factors. Misdiagnosing endogenous eczema for contact dermatitis is a major cause of chronicity. Often there is a multifactorial aetiology and iatrogenic sensitization may aggravate the clinical picture. The elimination of the causative agent is absolutely essential.[2] All other efforts only treat symptoms, but do not address the cause of contact dermatitis.

The mainstay of the symptomatic treatment of chronic contact dermatitis is still topical steroids.[3] Mid- and low-potency steroids are usually applied on a daily or twice-daily basis. Occlusive treatment is desirable, e.g. using a plastic wrap covering a steroid-containing cream or ointment for 8–10h/day, because it improves the penetration of the drug into the skin.[4] High potency steroids may be used for flares, but once dermatitis is controlled the potency should be tapered ("step therapy"). By alternatively applying steroids and ointments containing urea or lactic acid ("tandem therapy") the quantity of steroids can be limited. Emollients should be used as often as possible. Generally, a liberal use of emollients will reduce the steroid requirement ("interval therapy").[5] With the appropriate use of steroids, tachyphylaxis can be avoided.

Hyperplastic areas can be treated by incorporating salicylic acid.[6] Very resistant plaques may resolve after intralesional injection of steroids.[7] Oral acitretin and topical calcipotriol are other options in an antiproliferative treatment.

Even the best treatment fails if an appropriate vehicle has not been selected. Localization of skin changes, the patient's skin type and the eczema stage have to be taken into consideration. Generally, the more chronic the eczema, the higher the lipid content of the treatment should be. Oil-based ointment formulations usually contain less preservative than cream-based ones. This becomes important when long-term treatment is required, to prevent contact dermatitis due to allergens present in the vehicle. Additionally, the cosmetic acceptability of the topical treatment is very important for patient compliance.

Tar ointments were the mainstay of therapy before topical steroids were introduced. Due to its anti-infiltrative, antipruriginous and antimicrobial qualities, coal tar still is an effective alternative to topical steroids. The increasing corticophobia of many patients has also contributed to its renaissance. In chronic eczema of irritant cause, it is even more effective than steroids.[8] Inflammatory disruption of the epidermal barrier permits bacterial overgrowth and impetiginization. Topical treatment with antibiotics or antiseptics may be required. Long-term colonization with, e.g. *Staphylococcus aureus*, may have an adverse effect on eczema, possibly by releasing superantigens. It is therefore worth considering reducing this colonization by using antiseptics.[9]

Tap-water iontophoresis reduces hyperhidrosis and is a supportive measure for dyshidrotic eczema of the hands or feet.

For patients with severe chronic eczema that is not controllable by topical treatment, local UV B and/or UV A irradiation can be beneficial.[10,11] Psoralen photochemotherapy (PUVA) is reported to have a good effect in chronic eczema.[12] As oral psoralen photochemotherapy has several drawbacks for the patient, local PUVA-bath or -cream therapy is a rather simple and effective procedure without immediate side-effects.[13] Superficial X-ray therapy is indicated only in extensively resistant circumscribed eczema, after all other therapy options have been exhausted and after consideration of the patient's age.

Interval systemic steroid therapy may lead to dramatic improvements. Nevertheless it has a number of disadvantages. Beside the multiple systemic side-effects, the relapse rate is high, with inflammation returning shortly after the medication is discontinued. The rapid clearing of eczema sometimes reduces the patient's interest in protracted topical treatment that has only slowly noticeable success.

On occasions when systemic corticosteroids have failed or have given rise to unacceptable side-effects, immunosuppressive drugs such as azathioprine, cyclophosphamide or cyclosporin A may be indicated.[14] Topical tacrolimus (FK-506) is gaining increasing interest in the treatment of chronic dermatitis.[15]

Stress may worsen eczematous conditions. Chronic eczema may prevent sleep and threaten employment, sanity and personal relationships. Psychological support can therefore be of great value. Sedative antihistamines reduce the itch and support sleep; these are best given at night. The therapeutic effect of diets in contact dermatitis is controversal. For haematogenous allergic contact eczema, i.e. nickel-induced, an allergen-eliminating diet may be useful. For irritant contact dermatitis there is no obvious benefit from any food modifications. Cigarette smoking is suspected to aggravate eczema.[16] Alternative therapies such as hypnotherapy, acupuncture, homeopathy or herbal medicine are increasingly being used. However, no proof of efficacy has been presented.

In chronic eczema, scratching may become habitual and is often done unconsciously, a fact that causes difficulties in eradicating the disease. Bandaging may stop the constant itch–scratch cycle. This can be done by using paste bandages or wet wraps. It is also recommended in cases where artificial "upkeep" of eczema is suspected.

Another reason for chronicity of contact dermatitis is a lack of patient cooperation. Success depends partly on the dermatologist's understanding of the patient's personality, domestic and social conditions and ability to carry out treatment satisfactorily. Hospitalization should be encouraged when the dermatologist is not satisfied that the aetiologic factors have been fully elucidated or when treatment can not be effectively carried out at home. Short but intensive hospital treatment may be more effective and cost saving than a protracted outpatient treatment with sick leave.

The goal of therapy should be explained to the patient as "controlling the problem". Support, understanding and education should be offered. Patients should be encouraged to practise good skin care daily and to treat flare-ups promptly.[9] A programme for avoiding contact with causative agents, such as irritants and allergens, should be carefully outlined to the patient. Advice should be given on how to protect the skin. As far as the hands are involved, rubber gloves with cotton liners should be worn when dealing with skin-challenging agents. Barrier creams have been proved to be effective as well.[17] Generally, affected skin should be washed infrequently using mild or superfatted synthetic cleansers (syndets). Regular use of basic emollients and moisturizers to counteract dryness is important.[18]

References

1. Rycroft RJG, The management of hand eczema. *The Practitioner* 1984; **228**:1019–1123.
2. Harnack K, Grundzüge der Ekzemtherapie. *Z Arztl Fortbild* 1990; **84**:1184–1186.
3. August PJ, The environmental causes and management of eczema. *The Practitioner* 1987; **231**:495–500.
4. Braun-Falco O, Plewig G, Wolff HH, Winkelmann RK, eds. *Dermatology*. Berlin: Springer; 1991:316–366.

5. Burg G, Elsner P, Hartmann AA, *Der Ekzempatient in der Praxis*. Berlin: De Gruyter; 1990:73–89.

6. Hersle K, Mobacken H, Hyperkeratotic dermatitis of the palms. *Br J Dermatol* 1982; **107**:145–202.

7. Epstein E, Hand dermatitis. Practical managemment and current concepts. *J Am Acad Dermatol* 1984; **10**:395–424.

8. Elsner P, Aktuelle Ekzemtherapie. *Akt Dermatol* 1998; **24**:377–381.

9. Zug KA, McKay M, Eczematous dermatitis: a practical review. *Am Fam Physician* 1996; **54**:1243–1250.

10. Sjövall P, Christensen OB, Local and systemic effect of UVB irradiation in patients with chronic hand eczema. *Acta Dermatol Venereol (Stockh)* 1987; **67**:538–541.

11. Schmidt T, Abeck D, Boeck K et al., UVA1 irradiation is effective in treatment of chronic vesicular dyshydrotic hand eczema. *Acta Dermatol Venereol* 1998; **78**:318–319.

12. Larkö O, Phototherapy of eczema. *Photodermatol Photoimmunol Photomed* 1996; **12**:91–94.

13. Schempp CM, Müller H, Czech W et al., Treatment of chronic palmoplantar eczema with local bath–PUVA therapy. *J Am Acad Dermatol* 1997; **36**:733–737.

14. Morrison JGL, Schulz EJ, Treatment of eczema with cyclophosphamide and azathioprine. *Br J Dermatol* 1978; **98**:203–207.

15. Ruzicka T, Bieber T, Schöpf E et al., A short-term trial of tacrolimus ointment for atopic dermatitis. *N Engl J Med* 1997; **337**:816–821.

16. Sprince NL, Palmer JA, Popendorf W et al., Dermatitis among automobile production machine operators exposed to metal-working fluids. *Am J Ind Med* 1996; **30**:421–429.

17. Wigger-Alberti W, Elsner P, Preventive measures in contact dermatitis. *Clin Dermatol* 1997; **15**:661–665.

18. Buxton PK, Treatment of eczema and inflammatory dermatoses. *Br Med J* 1987; **295**:1112–1114.

21. Sources of Patch Test Materials

Matthias Gebhardt

Patch test allergens

Patch test allergens can be ordered from the following providers:

Chemotechnique Diagnostics

PO Box 80, Edvard Ols väg 2, S-230 42 Tygelsjö, Malmö, Sweden.
Phone: +46 40 46 60 77. Fax: +46 40 46 67 00
e-mail: info@chemotechnique.se. Homepage: www.chemotechnique.se

For information about Chemotechnique products in North America contact:
Dormer Laboratories, Inc., 91 Kelfield Street #5, Rexdale, Ontario M9W 5A3, Canada.
Phone: +1 416 242 6167. Fax: +1 416 242 9487

Hermal

Hermal is a company of the Boots Healthcare International Group:
Hermal Kurt Herrmann GmbH & Co, Scholtzstrasse 3, D-21465 Reinbek, Germany.
Phone: +49 40 7 27 04 0. Fax: +49 40 7 22 92 96
e-mail: info@hermal.de

Trolab

Trolab is contactable at the same address as Hermal. Its products are imported to and distributed in North America by:
Omniderm Inc., 997 Seguin, Hudson, Quebec J0P 1H0, Canada.
Phone: +1 514 458 0158.

TRUE Test

Information about using and ordering TRUE Test can be obtained at 1-800-TRUETEST. It is manufactured by Pharmacia & Upjohn Hillerød A/S, Denmark.

Distribution in the USA, Latin America, Asia Pacific, Eastern Europe, Middle East, Africa is by:
Glaxo Wellcome Inc., Research Triangle Park, North Carolina 27709, USA.
Homepage: www.truetest.com

Glaxo Wellcome have the rights to TRUE Test in all the countries mentioned above. While it is currently not available in these markets (except for the USA), the company is planning to register it in major markets in these regions during 1998. In the meantime specific requests can be addressed to:

HVD Vertriebsgesellschaft mbH, Wurzbachgasse 18, A-1152, Austria.
Phone: +43 1 982 9509. Fax: +43 1 982 1317

In Japan, True Test is not yet available but in future it will be available from:

Sato Pharmaceutical Co. Ltd, 5-27 1-chome, Motoakasaka, Minato-Ku, Tokyo 107, Japan.
Phone. +81 3 5412 7342. Fax: +81 3 5412 7332

In Western Europe, Australia/New Zealand:

ALK-Abello, Bøge Alle 10-12, DK-2970 Hørsholm, Denmark.
Phone: +45 45 76 77 77. Fax: +45 45 74 89 39

Brial Allergen GmbH

Alte Münsterstraße 10, D-48268 Greven, Germany.
Phone: +49 2571 9397 0. Fax: +49 2571 9397 20

The German company has a network of European distributors for patch test substances:

Germany	HAL Allergie GmbH, Kölner Landstraße 34a, D-40591 Düsseldorf
The Netherlands	HAL Allergen Laboratorium B.V., Gonnetstraat 26, NL-2011 KA Haarlem
Belgium	HALAB Allergy Service, Rue Antoine Nysstraat 86, B-1070 Brussels
France	ISOTEC, 10, Avenue Ampere B.P. 220, F-78051 St Quentin Cedex
Italy	Laboratorio Farmaceutica Lofarma, Viale Cassala 40, I-20143 Milano
Austria	Epipharm, Bannerstrasse 10, A-4060 Linz
Switzerland	E.E. Isler-Ernst, MD Allergy Service International, Steinbrüchelstrasse 14, CH-8053 Zurich, or Teomed AG, Schwamendingenstrasse 122, CH-8062 Zurich
UK	Allerayde Ltd, 3 Sanigar Court, Whittle Close, Newark, Notts, NG24 2BW
Turkey	Alser Asi, Serum Ve Tibbi Cihazlar, San. Ve Ticaret LTD. STI, Tunali Hilmi Cd. Bugday Sk. 6/42, 06700 Kavaklidere-Ankara, or ALMED, AstimAllergji Ilac, San. Ve Ticaret LTD. STI, Tuglacibasi Mah. Kayisdagi Cad. No. 134/9, Götztepe-Istanbul

TRUE Test Allergens

Patch	Allergen	Concentration (μg/cm²)
Panel 1		
1.	Nickel sulphate	200
2.	Wool alcohols	1000
3.	Neomycin sulphate	230
4.	Potassium dichromate	23
5.	Caine mix	630
6.	Fragrance mix	430
7.	Colophony BP	850
8.	Epoxy resin	50
9.	Quinoline mix	190
10.	Balsam of Peru	800
11.	Ethylenediaminedihydrochloride	50
12.	Cobalt chloride	20
Panel 2		
13.	*p*-tert-Butylphenol formaldehyde resin	40
14.	Parabens mix	1000
15.	Carba mix	250
16.	Black rubber mix (PPD-mix)	75
17.	Cl+Me-Isothiazolinone (Kathon CG)	4
18.	Quaternium-15	100
19.	Mercaptobenzothiazole	75
20.	Paraphenylenediamine	90
21.	Formaldehyde	180
22.	Mercapto mix	75
23.	Thiomersal	8
24.	Thiuram mix	25

Hermal / Trolab Allergens

Serial no.	Substance	Concentration (%)	Art. no.
European standard (ES)			
1.	Potassium dichromate	0.5	E 0001
2.	Neomycin sulphate	20	E 0010
3.	Thiuram mix	1	E 0023
4.	Paraphenylenediamine free base	1	E 0034
5.	Cobalt chloride, $6H_2O$	1	E 0002
6.	Benzocaine	5	E 0011
7.	Formaldehyde (in water)	1	E 0004
8.	Colophony	20	E 0017
9.	Clioquinol	5	E 0015
10.	Balsam of Peru	25	E 0008

Serial no.	*Substance*	*Concentration (%)*	*Art. no.*
11.	*N*-Isopropyl-*N'*-phenyl paraphenylenediamine	0.1	E 1004
12.	Wool alcohols	30	E 0020
13.	Mercapto mix	1	E 0025
14.	Epoxy resin	1	E 0021
15.	Paraben mix	16	E 2469
16.	*p*-tert-butylphenol formaldehyde resin	1	E 0030
17.	Fragrance mix	8	E 0029
18.	Quaternium-15	1	E 0031
19.	Nickel sulphate, $6H_2O$	5	E 0003
20.	5-Chloro-2-methyl-4-isothiazolin-3-one + 2-methyl-4-isothiazolin-3-one (3:1 in water)	0.01	E 0115
21.	Mercaptobenzothiazole	2	E 1010
22.	Sesquiterpene lactone mix	0.1	E 2459
23.	Primin (important in only some countries)	0.01	E 0032

Antimicrobials, preservatives, antioxidants (AP)

Technical use mainly			
1.	1,3,5-Tris(2-hydroxyethyl)-hexahydrotriazine	1	E 0119
2.	Benzylhemiformal	1	E 2450
3.	Benzotriazole	1	E 0159
4.	1,2-Benzisothiazolin-3-one, sodium salt	0.1	E 2471
5.	Dibromodicyanobutane	0.3	E 2516
Cosmetic and medical use mainly			
6.	Chlorocresol	1	E 0105
7.	Chloroxylenol	1	E 0106
8.	Bronopol	0.5	E 0107
9.	Imidazolidinyl urea (Germall 115)	2	E 0109
10.	Phenylmercuric acetate	0.05	E 2502
11.	Sorbic acid	2	E 0113
12.	Chlorhexidine digluconate (in water)	0.5	E 0114
13.	Chloracetamide	0.2	E 0117
14.	Glutar(di)aldehyde	0.3	E 2498
15.	Thiomersal	0.1	E 0600
16.	Chlorquinaldol	5	E 0104
17.	Benzalkonium chloride	0.1	E 2339
18.	Triclosan	2	E 0158
19.	Diazolidinyl urea (Germall II)	2	E 2386
20.	Dibromodicyanobutane/phenoxyethanol (1:4)	1	E 2515
21.	DMDM Hydantoin (in water)	2	E 2476
22.	Phenoxyethanol	1	E 2392
23.	Sodium metabisulphite	1	E 2412
24.	Cetylpyridinium chloride	0.1	E 2315
25.	Glyoxal trimer (dihydrate)	1	E 2517
Antioxidants			
26.	Butylhydroxytoluene	2	E 0110
27.	Butylhydroxyanisole	2	E 0111

Serial no.	Substance	Concentration (%)	Art. no.
28.	Dodecyl gallate (lauryl gallate)	0.3	E 2496
29.	tert-Butylhydroquinone	1	E 2434
30.	Propyl gallate	0.5	E 2497
31.	Octyl gallate	0.3	E 2495
Cosmetics (COS)			
1.	Hydroquinone	1	E 0800
2.	Toluenesulphonamide formaldehyde resin	10	E 0908
3.	Abitol®	10	E 0915
4.	Compositae mix	6	E 2369
5.	Benzyl salicylate	1	E 1102
6.	Vanillin	10	E 1310
7.	Lemon grass oil	2	E 1355
8.	Balsam of Tolu	20	E 1652
9.	Cocamidopropylbetaine (in water)	1	E 2303
10.	Abietic acid	10	E 2382
11.	Sodium benzoate	5	E 2385
12.	Benzyl alcohol	1	E 2388
13.	Dexpanthenol	5	E 2387
Dental materials (DM)			
1.	Menthol	1	E 2304
2.	Peppermint oil	2	E 1358
3.	Benzoyl peroxide	1	E 0201
4.	Hydroquinone	1	E 0800
5.	Bisphenol A	1	E 0965
6.	Methyl methacrylate	2	E 1800
7.	*N,N*-Dimethyl-*p*-toluidine	2	E 0963
8.	Ethyleneglycol dimethacrylate	2	E 1850
9.	Triethyleneglycol dimethacrylate	2	E 1851
10.	BIS-GMA	2	E 1852
11.	Diurethane dimethacrylate	2	E 2475
12.	(2-Hydroxyethyl) methacrylate (2-HEMA)	1	E 2477
13.	Eugenol	1	E 1302
14.	Ammoniated mercury	1	E 0602
15.	Potassium dicyanoaurate (in water)	0.002	E 0605
16.	Sodium thiosulphatoaurate	0.25	E 2507
17.	Palladium chloride	1	E 0651
18.	Ammonium tetrachloroplatinate	0.25	E 0650
19.	Amalgam	5	E 2509
20.	Amalgam alloying metals	20	E 2508
Hairdressing (HD)			
1.	*p*-Toluenediamine	1	E 0308
2.	Glyceryl monothioglycolate	1	E 0311
3.	Ammonium thioglycolate	1	E 0309
4.	Ammonium persulphate	2.5	E 0306

Serial no.	Substance	Concentration (%)	Art. no.
5.	4-Aminophenol	1	E 2302
6.	3-Aminophenol	1	E 2301

Medicaments (ME)

Serial no.	Substance	Concentration (%)	Art. no.
Miscellaneous			
1.	Benzoyl peroxide	1	E 0201
2.	Phenyl salicylate	1	E 2100
3.	Ethylenediamine dihydrochloride	1	E 0027
4.	Bufexamac	5	E 2395
5.	Propolis	10	E 1207
Antibiotics, antiseptics and antimycotics			
6.	Bacitracin	20	E 2151
7.	Chloramphenicol	5	E 2152
8.	Gentamycin sulphate	20	E 2154
9.	Kanamycin sulphate	10	E 2313
10.	Tetracycline hydrochloride	2	E 2306
11.	Sulphanilamide	5	E 2160
12.	Nystatin	2	E 2491
13.	Erythromycin	1	E 2499
14.	Chlorquinaldol	5	E 0104
15.	Fusidic acid sodium salt	2	E 2454
16.	Clotrimazole	5	E 2389
17.	Oxytetracycline	3	E 2416
Local anaesthetics			
18.	Cinchocaine hydrochloride	5	E 0401
19.	Tetracaine (amethocaine) hydrochloride	1	E 0402
20.	Lidocaine hydrochloride	15	E 0403
21.	Polidocanol	3	E 2501
Corticosteroids[a]			
22.	Amcinonide	0.1	E 2481
23.	Betamethasone-17-valerate	0.12	E 2482
24.	Clobetasol-17-propionate	0.25	E 2483
25.	Hydrocortisone	1	E 2484
26.	Hydrocortisone-17-butyrate	0.1	E 2485
27.	Triamcinolone acetonide	0.1	E 2486
28.	Budesonide	0.1	E 2504
29.	Prednisolone	1	E 2505
Ophthalmics			
30.	Atropine sulphate (in water)	1	E 2415
31.	Edetic acid disodium salt	1	E 2384
32.	Phenylephrine hydrochloride (in water)	10	E 2414
33.	Pilocarpine hydrochloride (in water)	1	E 2407
34.	Polymyxin B sulphate	3	E 2437

[a]According to the results of the German Contact Dermatitis Group.

Serial no.	Substance	Concentration (%)	Art. no.
Metal compounds (MC)			
1.	Ammoniated mercury	1	E 0602
2.	Potassium dicyanoaurate (in water)	0.002	E 0605
3.	Sodium thiosulphatoaurate	0.25	E 2507
4.	Ammonium tetrachloroplatinate	0.25	E 0650
5.	Palladium chloride	1	E 0651
Metalworking and technical oils (MW)			
1.	Benzylhemiformal	1	E 2450
2.	Chloroxylenol	1	E 0106
3.	Bronopol	0.5	E 0107
4.	Chloracetamide	0.2	E 0117
5.	1,3,5-Tris(2-hydroxyethyl)-hexahydrotriazine	1	E 0119
6.	Bioban® CS-1246	1	E 2422
7.	Triclosan	2	E 0158
8.	Benzotriazole	1	E 0159
9.	Monoethanolamine	2	E 2445
10.	*p*-tert Butylcatechol	1	E 0918
11.	Trolamine (triethanolamine)	2.5	E 1701
12.	Amerchol® L 101	50	E 1750
13.	Dipentene (DL-Limonene)	2	E 2000
14.	Dichlorophene	0.5	E 2316
15.	Propyleneglycol	5	E 2323
16.	Diethanolamine	2	E 2401
17.	2-Hydroxymethyl-2-nitro-1,3-propanediol	1	E 2410
18.	Bioban® CS-1135	1	E 2420
19.	Coconut diethanolamide	0.5	E 2424
20.	Bioban® P-1487	1	E 2426
21.	Octylisothiazolinone	0.025	E 2427
22.	Methylene-bis(methyloxazolidine)	1	E 2452
23.	Dibromodicyanobutane	0.3	E 2516
24.	1,2-Benzisothiazolin-3-one, sodium salt	0.1	E 2471
25.	Abietic acid	10	E 2382
Perfumes and flavourings (PF)			
1.	Benzyl salicylate	1	E 1102
2.	Clove oil	2	E 1308
3.	Orange oil	2	E 1309
4.	Vanillin	10	E 1310
5.	Benzaldehyde	5	E 1350
6.	Benzylcinnamate	5	E 1351
7.	Cedarwood oil	10	E 1352
8.	Eucalyptus oil	2	E 1353
9.	Laurel oil	2	E 1354
10.	Lemon grass oil	2	E 1355
11.	Lemon oil	2	E 1356

Serial no.	Substance	Concentration (%)	Art. no.
12.	Neroli oil	2	E 1357
13.	Peppermint oil	2	E 1358
14.	Salicylaldehyde	2	E 1359

Photoallergens[b] (PA)

1.	Tetrachloro salicylanilide	0.1	E 0102
2.	5-Bromo-4'-chlorosalicylanilide	1	E 2354
3.	Hexachlorophene	1	E 0101
4.	Bithionol	1	E 0100
5.	Sulphanilamide	5	E 2160
6.	Promethazine hydrochloride	0.1	E 2356
7.	Quinidine sulphate	1	E 2358
8.	Musk ambrette	5	E 2203
9.	Fragrance mix	8	E 0029
10.	p-Aminobenzoic acid	10	E 2359
11.	2-Ethylhexyl-*p*-dimethylaminobenzoate	10	E 2365
12.	Benzophenone 4	10	E 2500
13.	4-tert-Butyl-4'-methoxy-dibenzoylmethane	10	E 2364
14.	Isoamyl-*p*-methoxycinnamate	10	E 2368
15.	2-Ethylhexyl-p-methoxycinnamate	10	E 2366
16.	3-(4-Methylbenzylidene)-camphor	10	E 2362
17.	2-Phenyl-5-benzimidazolsulphonic acid	10	E 2367
18.	Oxybenzone	10	E 2361
Annexe			
19.	Tribromsalan	1	E 0103
20.	Chlorpromazine hydrochloride	0.1	E 2201
21.	Thiourea	0.1	E 2255
22.	Olaquindox	1	E 2494

[b]According to the results of a cooperative photopatch test study conducted by 45 dermatological centres in Austria, Germany and Switzerland.

Photographic chemicals (PC)

1.	Ammonium persulphate	2.5	E 0306
2.	*p*-Methylaminophenol sulphate (Metol)	1	E 0801
3.	Colour Developer CD 2	1	E 0803
4.	Colour Developer CD 3	1	E 0804
5.	Colour Developer CD 4	1	E 0806
6.	1-Phenyl-3-pyrazolidinone (Phenidone)	1	E 0809
7.	Pyrogallol	1	E 0350
8.	4-Aminophenol	1	E 2302
9.	Hydroquinone	1	E 0800
10.	Triphenyl phosphate	5	E 0959

Plants (PL)

1.	Dipentene (DL-Limonene)	2	E 2000
2.	Usnic acid	0.1	E 2052

Serial no.	Substance	Concentration (%)	Art. no.
3.	Tansy extract	1	E 2439
4.	Arnica extract	0.5	E 2441
5.	Feverfew flower extract	1	E 2503
6.	Chamomile extract	2.5	E 2408
7.	Yarrow extract	1	E 2440
Plastics and glues (PG)			
Miscellaneous			
1.	Phenol formaldehyde resin (Novolac)	5	E 0901
2.	Phenol formaldehyde resin (Resol)	5	E 0911
3.	Abitol®	10	E 0915
4.	Benzoyl peroxide	1	E 0201
5.	Turpentine oil	10	E 2322
6.	Hydroquinone	1	E 0800
7.	*p*-tert-Butylphenol	1	E 0920
8.	*N,N*-Dimethyl-*p*-toluidine	2	E 0963
Epoxies			
9.	Triethylenetetramine	0.5	E 0905
10.	4-4'-Diaminodiphenylmethane	0.5	E 0906
11.	Diethylenetriamine	0.5	E 0913
12.	Isophoronediamine	0.5	E 0914
13.	Hexamethylenetetramine	1	E 2318
14.	Cresylglycidylether	0.25	E 0917
15.	Bisphenol A	1	E 0965
Plasticizer			
16.	Di-n-Butylphthalate	5	E 0903
17.	Tricresyl phosphate (isomer blend)	5	E 2511
18.	Triphenyl phosphate	5	E 0959
19.	Dimethylphthalate	5	E 0954
20.	Di-2-Ethylhexyl-phthalate	5	E 0960
Isocyanates			
21.	Diphenylmethane-4,4-diisocyanate	1	E 2513
22.	Toluenediisocyanate	1	E 2514
Acrylates			
23.	(2-Hydroxyethyl) methacrylate (2-HEMA)	1	E 2477
24.	Methyl methacrylate	2	E 1800
25.	Ethyleneglycol dimethacrylate	2	E 1850
26.	Triethyleneglycol dimethacrylate	2	E 1851
27.	BIS-GMA	2	E 1852
28.	Diurethane dimethacrylate	2	E 2475
Rubber chemicals (RC)			
1.	Hexamethylenetetramine	1	E 2318

Serial no.	Substance	Concentration (%)	Art. no.
2.	Diphenylthiourea	1	E 1021
3.	Dibutylthiourea	1	E 1025
4.	1,3-Diphenylguanidine	1	E 1002
5.	Bis(diethyldithiocarbamato) zinc	1	E 1009
6.	*N,N'*-Diphenylparaphenylenediamine	0.25	E 1013
7.	Bis(dibutyldithiocarbamato) zinc	1	E 1019
8.	Cyclohexylthiophthalimide	1	E 1051
9.	Phenyl-β-naphthylamine	1	E 2409
Sunscreen Agents (SA)			
1.	2-Phenyl-5-benzimidazolsulphonic acid (Eusolex® 232)	10	E 2367
2.	4-tert-Butyl-4'-methoxy-dibenzoylmethane (Parsol® 1789)	10	E 2364
3.	*p*-Aminobenzoic acid (PABA)	10	E 2359
4.	2-Ethylhexyl-p-dimethylaminobenzoate (Escalol® 507)	10	E 2365
5.	2-Ethylhexyl-*p*-methoxycinnamate (Parsol® MCX)	10	E 2366
6.	3-(4-Methylbenzylidene)-camphor (Eusolex® 6300)	10	E 2362
7.	Oxybenzone (Eusolex® 4360)	10	E 2361
8.	Isoamyl-*p*-methoxycinnamate	10	E 2368
9.	Benzophenone 4	10	E 2500
Textile and leather dyes (TD)			
1.	Disperse orange 3	1	E 0502
2.	Disperse yellow 3	1	E 0503
3.	Disperse red 1	1	E 0504
4.	Disperse red 17	1	E 0505
5.	Disperse blue 3	1	E 0506
6.	Disperse red 11	1	E 2478
7.	Disperse yellow 9	1	E 2479
8.	Disperse blue 1	1	E 2473
9.	Naphthol AS	1	E 2474
10.	4-Aminophenol	1	E 2302
11.	4-Aminoazobenzene	1	E 2435
12.	Acid yellow 36	1	E 2403
13.	Bismark brown R	0.5	E 2428
14.	Disperse blue mix (124/106)	1	E 2512
Vehicles and emulsifiers (VE)			
1.	Trolamine (triethanolamine)	2.5	E 1701
2.	Propyleneglycol	5	E 2323
3.	Sorbitan sesquioleate	20	E 1703
4.	Cetyl/stearyl alcohol	20	E 1704
5.	Amerchol® L101	50	E 1750

6.	Polyethylene glycol ointment	100	E 2337
7.	Isopropyl myristate	10	E 2336
Miscellaneous (MIC)			
1.	Hexylresorcinol	0.25	E 0312
2.	Potassium dichromate	0.25	E 2506
3.	Propyleneglycol (in water)	20	E 2472
Constituents of the fragrance mix			
	Cinnamyl alcohol	1	E 1300
	Cinnamaldehyde	1	E 1301
	Eugenol	1	E 1302
	α-Amyl-cinnamaldehyde	1	E 1303
	Hydroxycitronellal	1	E 1304
	Geraniol	1	E 1305
	Isoeugenol	1	E 1306
	Oak moss absolute	1	E 1307
	Sorbitan sesquioleate	20	E 1703
Constituents of the thiuram mix			
	Tetramethylthiuram disulphide	0.25	E 1011
	Tetraethylthiuram disulphide	0.25	E 1016
	Tetramethylthiuram monosulphide	0.25	E 1008
	Dipentamethylenethiuram disulphide	0.25	E 1017
Constituents of the mercapto mix			
	Dibenzothiazyl disulphide	1	E 1014
	N-Cyclohexylbenzothiazyl sulphenamide	1	E 1000
	Morpholinylmercaptobenzothiazole	0.5	E 1015
Constituents of the parabens mix			
	Methylparahydroxybenzoate	3	E 0151
	Ethylparahydroxybenzoate	3	E 0152
	Propylparahydroxybenzoate	3	E 0153
	Butylparahydroxybenzoate	3	E 0154
Control (C)			
1.	White petrolatum	100	E 8999

Chemotechnique Allergens

European standard (ES)[a]			
1.	Potassium dichromate	0.5 pet	P014
2.	4-Phenylenediamine base	1.0 pet	P006
3.	Thiuram mix:	1.0 pet	Mx01
	Tetramethylthiuram monosulphide (TMTM)	0.25	T006

Serial no.	Substance	Concentration (%)	Art. no.
	Teramethylthiuram disulphide (TMTD)	0.25	T005
	Tetraethylthiuram disulphide (TETD)	0.25	T002
	Dipentamethylenethiuram disulphide (PTD)	0.25	D019
4.	Neomycin sulphate	20.0 pet	N001
5.	Cobalt chloride	1.0 pet	C017
6.	Benzocaine	5.0 pet	B004
7.	Nickel sulphate	5.0 pet	N002
8.	Quinoline mix:	6.0 pet	Mx02
	Clioquinol	3.0	C015
	Chlorquinaldol	3.0	C012
9.	Colophony	20.0 pet	C020
10.	Parabens:	12.0 pet	Mx03
	Methyl-4-hydroxybenzoate	3.0	M012
	Ethyl-4-hydroxybenzoate	3.0	E010
	Propyl-4-hydroxybenzoate	3.0	P020
	Butyl-4-hydroxybenzoate	3.0	B020
11.	*N*-Isopropyl-*N*-phenyl-4-phenylenediamine	0.1 pet	I004
12.	Wool alcohols	30.0 pet	W001
13.	Mercapto mix:	2.0 pet	Mx05
	N-cyclohexylbenzothiazyl sulphenamide	0.5	C023
	Mercaptobenzothiazole	0.5	M003
	Dibenzothiazyl disulphide	0.5	D003
	Morpholinylmercaptobenzothiazole	0.5	M016
14.	Epoxy resin	1.0 pet	E002
15.	Balsam of Peru	25.0 pet	B001
16.	4-tert-Butylphenol formaldehyde resin	1.0 pet	B024
17.	Mercaptobenzothiazole (MBT)	2.0 pet	M003
18.	Formaldehyde	1.0 aq	F002
19.	Fragrance mix:[b]	8.0 pet	Mx07
	Cinnamic alcohol	1.0	C013
	Cinnamic aldehyde	1.0	C014
	Hydroxycitronellal	1.0	H008
	Amylcinnamaldehyde	1.0	A014
	Geraniol	1.0	G001
	Eugenol	1.0	E016
	Isoeugenol	1.0	I002
	Oakmoss absolute	1.0	O001
20.	Sesquiterpene lactone mix:	0.1 pet	Mx18
	Alantolactone	0.033	A003
	Dehydrocostus lactone + costunolide	0.067	
21.	Quaternium 15 (Dowicil 200)	1.0 pet	C007
22.	Primin	0.01 pet	M008
23.	Cl+Me-isothiazolinone (Kathon CG,100 ppm)	0.01 aq	C009

[a]Revised May 1993.

[b]Emulsifier: Sorbitan sesquioleate 5%.

Various national standard series, developed by the national contact dermatitis research groups, are also available on request.

Serial no.	Substance	Concentration (%)	Art. no.
Bakery series			
1.	Vanillin	10.0 pet	V001
2.	Eugenol	2.0 pet	E016
3.	Isoeugenol	2.0 pet	I002
4.	Sodium benzoate	5.0 pet	S001
5.	2,6-ditert-Butyl-4-cresol (BHT)	2.0 pet	D006
6.	Menthol	2.0 pet	M002
7.	Cinnamic alcohol	2.0 pet	C013
8.	Cinnamic aldehyde	1.0 pet	C014
9.	2-tert-Butyl-4-methoxyphenol (BHA)	2.0 pet	B022
10.	Anethole	5.0 pet	A015
11.	Sorbic acid	2.0 pet	S003
12.	Benzoic acid	5.0 pet	B005
13.	Propionic acid	3.0 pet	P018
14.	Octyl gallate	0.25 pet	O002
15.	Dipentene (Limonene)	1.0 pet	D020
16.	Ammonium persulphate	2.5 pet	A011
17.	Benzoylperoxide	1.0 pet	B007
18.	Propyl gallate	1.0 pet	P021
19.	Dodecyl gallate	0.25 pet	D042
Corticosteroid series[c]			
1.	Budesonide	0.1 pet	B033
2.	Betamethasone-17-valerate	1.0 pet	B031
3.	Triamcinolone acetonide	1.0 pet	T030
4.	Tixocortol-21-pivalate	1.0 pet	T031
5.	Alclomethasone-17,21-dipropionate	1.0 pet	A023
6.	Clobetasol-17-propionate	1.0 pet	C028
7.	Dexamethasone-21-phosphate disodium salt	1.0 pet	D046
8.	Hydrocortisone-17-butyrate	1.0 alc	H021

[c]New August 1992.

Serial no.	Substance	Concentration (%)	Art. no.
Cosmetic series			
1.	Isopropyl myristate	20.0 pet	I003
2.	Amerchol L 101	50 pet	A004
3.	Triethanolamine	2.0 pet	T016
4.	Polyoxyethylenesorbitan mono-oleate (Tween 80)	5.0 pet	P013
5.	Sorbitan mono-oleate (Span 80)	5.0 pet	S004
6.	2-tert-Butyl-4-methoxyphenol (BHA)	2.0 pet	B022
7.	2,6-ditert-Butyl-4-cresol (BHT)	2.0 pet	D006
8.	Octyl gallate	0.25 pet	O002
9.	Triclosan (Irgasan DP 300)	2.0 pet	T014
10.	Sorbic acid	2.0 pet	S003
11.	4-Chloro-3-cresol (PCMC)	1.0 pet	C008
12.	4-Chloro-3-xylenol (PCMX)	0.5 pet	C010

Serial no.	Substance	Concentration (%)	Art. no.
13.	Thimerosal (Merthiolate)	0.1 pet	T007
14.	Imidazolidinylurea (Germall 115)	2.0 pet	I001
15.	Hexamethylenetetramine (Hexamin)	2.0 pet	H003
16.	Chlorhexidine digluconate	0.5 aq	C005
17.	Parabens[d]	12.0 pet	Mx03
18.	Phenylmercuric acetate	0.01 aq	P008
19.	Chloroacetamide	0.2 pet	C006
20.	Hexahydro-1,3,5-tris(hydroxyethyl)triazine (Grotan BK)	1.0 aq	H002
21.	Clioquinol (5-chloro-7-iodo-quinolinol)	5.0 pet	C015
22.	Ethylenediamine dihydrochloride	1.0 pet	E005
23.	Abitol	10.0 pet	A002
24.	Phenyl salicylate (Salol)	1.0 pet	P011
25.	2-Hydroxy-4-methoxybenzophenone	2.0 pet	H014
26.	Sorbitan sesquioleate	20.0 pet	S005
27.	Propyleneglycol	5.0 pet	P019
28.	Stearyl alcohol	30.0 pet	S006
29.	Cetyl alcohol	5.0 pet	C003
30.	Benzyl salicylate	2.0 pet	B010
31.	2-Bromo-2-nitropropane-1,3-diol (Bronopol)	0.25 pet	B015
32.	Sodium-2-pyridinethiol-1-oxide (Sodiumomadine)	0.1 aq	S002
33.	Cocamidopropyl betaine	1.0 aq	C018
34.	Benzyl alcohol	1.0 pet	B008
35.	Cl+Me-isothiazolinone (Kathon CG, 200 ppm)	0.02 aq	C009B
36.	tert-Butylhydroquinone	1.0 pet	B028
37.	2(2-Hydroxy-5-methylphenyl)benzotriazol (Tinuvin P)	1.0 pet	H016
38.	Propyl gallate	1.0 pet	P021
39.	Dodecyl gallate	0.25 pet	D042
40.	Quaternium 15 (Dowicil 200)[d]	1.0 pet	C007
41.	2-Phenoxyethanol	1.0 pet	P025
42.	Diazolidinylurea (Germall II)	2.0 pet	D044
43.	Euxyl K 400	0.5 pet	Mx17
44.	DMDM Hydantoin	2.0 aq	D047
45.	1,2-Dibromo-2,4-dicyanobutane	0.3 pet	D049

[d]Also present in standard series. Revised March 1998.

Dental screening[e]

1.	Methyl methacrylate	2.0 pet	M013
2.	Triethyleneglycol dimethacrylate	2.0 pet	T018
3.	Urethane dimethacrylate	2.0 pet	U004
4.	Ethyleneglycol dimethacrylate	2.0 pet	E007
5.	BIS-GMA	2.0 pet	H013
6.	*N,N*-Dimethyl-4-toluidine	5.0 pet	D016
7.	2-Hydroxy-4-methoxy-benzophenone	2.0 pet	H014

Serial no.	*Substance*	*Concentration (%)*	*Art. no.*
8.	1,4-Butanediol dimethacrylate	2.0 pet	B017
9.	BIS-MA	2.0 pet	M007
10.	Potassium dichromate[f]	0.5 pet	P014
11.	Mercury	0.5 pet	M005
12.	Cobalt chloride[f]	1.0 pet	C017
13.	2-Hydroxyethylmethacrylate	2.0 pet	H010
14.	Goldsodiumthiosulphate	0.5 pet	G005
15.	Nickel sulphate[f]	5.0 pet	N002
16.	Eugenol	2.0 pet	E016
17.	Colophony[f]	20.0 pet	C020
18.	*N*-Ethyl-4-toluenesulphonamide	0.1 pet	E015
19.	Formaldehyde[f]	1.0 aq	F002
20.	4-Tolyldiethanolamine	2.0 pet	T011
21.	Copper sulphate	2.0 pet	C022
22.	Methylhydroquinone	1.0 pet	M025
23.	Palladium chloride	2.0 pet	P001
24.	Aluminum chloride hexahydrate	2.0 pet	A022
25.	Camphoroquinone	1.0 pet	C026
26.	*N,N*-Dimethylaminoethyl methacrylate	0.2 pet	D045
27.	1,6-Hexanediol diacrylate	0.1 pet	H004
28.	2(2-Hydroxy-5-methylphenyl)benzotriazol	1.0 pet	H016
29.	Tetrahydrofurfuryl methacrylate	2.0 pet	T027
30.	Tin	50.0 pet	T008

[e]Revised May 1993.

[f]Also present in standard series.

Epoxy series[g]

1.	Hexamethylenetetramine	2.0 pet	H003
2.	Diaminodiphenylmethane	0.5 pet	D001
3.	Triethylenetetramine	0.5 pet	T019
4.	Phenylglycidylether	0.25 pet	P023
5.	Diethylenetriamine	1.0 pet	D010
6.	Isophorone diamine	0.1 pet	I006
7.	Epoxy resin, cycloaliphatic	0.5 pet	E020
8.	Ethylenediamine dihydrochloride	1.0 pet	E005

≠gRevised May 1990.

Fragrance series[h]

1.	Cinnamic aldehyde	1.0 pet	C014
2.	Cinnamic alcohol	2.0 pet	C013
3.	Amylcinnamaldehyde	2.0 pet	A014
4.	Eugenol	2.0 pet	E016
5.	Isoeugenol	2.0 pet	I002
6.	Geraniol	2.0 pet	G001
7.	Oakmoss absolute	2.0 pet	O001
8.	Hydroxycitronellal	2.0 pet	H008
9.	Narcissus absolute	2.0 pet	N006

Serial no.	Substance	Concentration (%)	Art. no.
10.	Musk xylene	1.0 pet	M021
11.	Musk tibetine	1.0 pet	M020
12.	Musk moskene	1.0 pet	M019
13.	Musk ketone	1.0 pet	M018
14.	Jasmine synthetic	2.0 pet	J001
15.	Benzyl salicylate	2.0 pet	B010
16.	Benzyl alcohol	1.0 pet	B008
17.	Vanillin	10.0 pet	V001
18.	Lavender absolute	2.0 pet	L001
19.	Cananga oil	2.0 pet	C002
20.	Rose oil, Bulgarian	2.0 pet	R003
21.	Ylang-Ylang oil	2.0 pet	Y001
22.	Geranium oil, Bourbon	2.0 pet	G002
23.	Jasmine absolute, Egyptian	2.0 pet	J002
24.	Sandalwood oil	2.0 pet	S009

[h]Revised October 1997.

Hairdressing series[i]

1.	4-Phenylenediamine base[j]	1.0 pet	P006
2.	2.5-Diaminotoluene sulphate	1.0 pet	D002
3.	2-Nitro-4-phenylenediamine	1.0 pet	N004
4.	Ammonium thioglycolate	2.5 aq	A012
5.	Ammonium persulphate	2.5 pet	A011
6.	Formaldehyde[j]	1.0 aq	F002
7.	Nickel sulphate[j]	5.0 pet	N002
8.	Cobalt chloride[j]	1.0 pet	C017
9.	Resorcinol	1.0 pet	R001
10.	3-Aminophenol	1.0 pet	A008
11.	4-Aminophenol	1.0 pet	A009
12.	Hydrogen peroxide	3.0 aq	H006
13.	Hydroquinone	1.0 pet	H007
14.	Balsam of Peru[j]	25.0 pet	B001
15.	Chloroacetamide	0.2 pet	C006
16.	Glyceryl monothioglycolate (GMTG)	1.0 pet	G004
17.	Cocamidopropylbetaine	1.0 aq	C018
18.	Cl+Me-isothiazolinone[j] (Kathon CG, 200 ppm)	0.02 aq	C009B
19.	2-Bromo-2-nitropropane-1,3-diol (Bronopol)	0.25 pet	B015
20.	Captan	0.5 pet	C025
21.	4-Chloro-3-cresol (PCMC)	1.0 pet	C008
22.	4-Chloro-3-xylenol (PCMX)	0.5 pet	C010
23.	Imidazolidinyl urea (Germall 115)	2.0 pet	I001
24.	Quaternium 15 (Dowicil 200)[j]	1.0 pet	C007
25.	Zinc pyrithione (Zinc omadine)	1.0 pet	Z006
26.	Diazolidinylurea (Germall II)	2.0 pet	D044

[i]Revised January 1996.

[j]Also present in standard series.

Serial no.	Substance	Concentration (%)	Art. no.
Isocyanate series[k]			
1.	Toluenediisocyanate (TDI)	2.0 pet	T009
2.	Diphenylmethane-4,4-diisocyanate (MDI)	2.0 pet	D023
3.	Diaminodiphenylmethane	0.5 pet	D001
4.	Isophoronediisocyanate (IPDI)	1.0 pet	I007
5.	Isophorone diamine (IPD)	0.1 pet	I006
6.	1,6-Hexamethylenediisocyanate (HDI)	0.1 pet	H022

[k]Revised May 1990.

Serial no.	Substance	Concentration (%)	Art. no.
Medicament series[l]			
1.	Chloramphenicol	5.0 pet	C032
2.	Kanamycin sulphate	10.0 pet	K001
3.	Quinine sulphate	1.0 pet	Q001
4.	Sulphanilamide	5.0 pet	S010
5.	Gentamicin sulphate	20.0 pet	G006
6.	Nitrofurazone	1.0 pet	N005
7.	Bacitracin	5.0 pet	B032
8.	Polymyxin B sulphate	5.0 pet	P026
9.	Caine mix III:	10.0 pet	Mx19
	Benzocaine	5.0 pet	
	Dibucaine–HCl (cinchocaine)	2.5 pet	
	Tetracaine–HCl (amethocaine)	2.5 pet	
10.	Miconazole	1.0 alc	M027
11.	Econazole nitrate	1.0 alc	E021
12.	Caine mix IV:	10.0 pet	Mx20
	Amylocaine hydrochloride	2.5 pet	
	Lignocaine (lidocaine)	5.0 pet	
	Prilocaine hydrochloride	2.5 pet	

[l]New August 1992.

Serial no.	Substance	Concentration (%)	Art. no.
(Meth) Acrylate series, adhesives, dental and other[m]			
1.	Methyl methacrylate	2.0 pet	M013
2.	n-Butyl methacrylate	2.0 pet	B021
3.	2-Hydroxyethyl methacrylate	2.0 pet	H010
4.	2-Hydroxypropyl methacrylate	2.0 pet	H018
5.	Ethyleneglycol dimethacrylate	2.0 pet	E007
6.	Triethyleneglycol dimethacrylate	2.0 pet	T018
7.	1,4-Butanediol dimethacrylate	2.0 pet	B017
8.	Urethane dimethacrylate	2.0 pet	U004
9.	BIS-MA	2.0 pet	M007
10.	BIS-GMA	2.0 pet	H013
11.	1,6-Hexanediol diacrylate	0.1 pet	H004
12.	Tetrahydrofurfuryl methacrylate	2.0 pet	T027
13.	Tetraethyleneglycol dimethacrylate	2.0 pet	T029
14.	*N,N*-Dimethylaminoethyl methacrylate	0.2 pet	D045

[m]Revised August 1992.

Serial no.	Substance	Concentration (%)	Art. no.
(Meth) Acrylate series and artificial nails[n]			
1.	Butyl acrylate	0.1 pet	B018
2.	Ethyl methacrylate	2.0 pet	E012
3.	n-Butyl methacrylate	2.0 pet	B021
4.	2-Hydroxyethyl methacrylate	2.0 pet	H010
5.	2-Hydroxypropyl methacrylate	2.0 pet	H018
6.	Ethyleneglycol dimethacrylate	2.0 pet	E007
7.	Triethyleneglycol dimethacrylate	2.0 pet	T018
8.	1,6-Hexanediol diacrylate	0.1 pet	H004
9.	Trimethylolpropane triacrylate	0.1 pet	T021
10.	Tetrahydrofurfuryl methacrylate	2.0 pet	T027
11.	Ethyl acrylate	0.1 pet	E004
12.	2-Hydroxyethyl acrylate	0.1 pet	H009
13.	Triethyleneglycol diacrylate	0.1 pet	T017

[n]Revised August 1992.

Serial no.	Substance	Concentration (%)	Art. no.
(Meth) Acrylate series and printing[o]			
1.	Ethyl acrylate	0.1 pet	E004
2.	2-Ethylhexyl acrylate	0.1 pet	E009
3.	2-Hydroxyethyl acrylate	0.1 pet	H009
4.	2-Hydroxypropyl acrylate	0.1 pet	H017
5.	Methyl methacrylate	2.0 pet	M013
6.	Ethyl methacrylate	2.0 pet	E012
7.	n-Butyl methacrylate	2.0 pet	B021
8.	2-Hydroxyethyl methacrylate	2.0 pet	H010
9.	2-Hydroxypropyl methacrylate	2.0 pet	H018
10.	Ethyleneglycol dimethacrylate	2.0 pet	E007
11.	Triethyleneglycol dimethacrylate	2.0 pet	T018
12.	BIS-EMA	1.0 pet	M006
13.	1,4-Butanediol diacrylate	0.1 pet	B016
14.	1,6-Hexanediol diacrylate	0.1 pet	H004
15.	Diethyleneglycol diacrylate	0.1 pet	D009
16.	Tripropyleneglycol diacrylate	0.1 pet	T023
17.	Trimethylolpropane triacrylate	0.1 pet	T021
18.	Pentaerythritol triacrylate	0.1 pet	P002
19.	Oligotriacrylate 480	0.1 pet	O003
20.	Epoxy acrylate	0.5 pet	E001
21.	Urethane diacrylate (aliphatic)	0.1 pet	U002
22.	Urethane diacrylate (aromatic)	0.05 pet	U003
23.	Triethyleneglycol diacrylate	0.1 pet	T017
24.	*N,N*-Methylenebisacrylamid	1.0 pet	M023

[o]Revised August 1992.

Serial no.	Substance	Concentration (%)	Art. no.
Oil and cooling fluid series[p]			
1.	Abietic acid	10.0 pet	A001
2.	4-Chloro-3-cresol (PCMC)	1.0 pet	C008
3.	4-Chloro-3-xylenol (PCMX)	0.5 pet	C010

Serial no.	Substance	Concentration (%)	Art. no.
4.	Dichlorophene	1.0 pet	D008
5.	2-Phenylphenol	1.0 pet	P010
6.	Propyleneglycol	5.0 pet	P019
7.	Triethanolamine	2.0 pet	T016
8.	4-tert-Butylbenzoic acid	1.0 pet	B019
9.	1,2-Benzisothiazolin-3-one	0.05 pet	B003
10.	Hexahydro-1,3,5-tris(hydroxyethyl)triazin	1.0 aq	H002
11.	Bioban P 1487	0.5 pet	E014
12.	Chloroacetamide	0.2 pet	C006
13.	*N*-Methylolchloroacetamide	0.1 pet	M014
14.	1H-Benzotriazol	1.0 pet	B006
15.	Ethylenediamine dihydrochloride	1.0 pet	E005
16.	Mercaptobenzothiazole	2.0 pet	M003
17.	Zinc ethylenebis(dithiocarbamate)	1.0 pet	Z005
18.	Triclosan (Irgasan DP 300)	2.0 pet	T014
19.	Bioban CS 1246	1.0 pet	A017
20.	Bioban CS 1135	1.0 pet	D015
21.	Tris nitro	1.0 pet	H015
22.	Thimerosal (Merthiolate)	0.1 pet	T007
23.	Hydrazine sulphate	1.0 pet	H005
24.	Trichlorocarbanilide (TCC)	1.0 pet	T013
25.	Formaldehyde[q]	1.0 aq	F002
26.	Amerchol L 101	50 pet	A004
27.	Dipentene (Limonene)	1.0 pet	D020
28.	Sodium-2-pyridinethiol-1-oxide	0.1 aq	S002
29.	2-Bromo-2-nitropropane-1,3-diol	0.25 pet	B015
30.	Coconut diethanolamide	0.5 pet	C019
31.	Cl+Me-isothiazolinone[q] (Kathon CG, 200 ppm)	0.02 aq	C009B
32.	Euxyl K 400	0.5 pet	Mx17
33.	2-n-Octyl-4-isothiazolin-3-one	0.1 pet	O004
34.	1,2-Dibromo-2,4-dicyanobutane	0.3 pet	D-049

[p]Revised March 1998.

[q]Also present in standard series.

Photographic chemicals series[r]

Serial no.	Substance	Concentration (%)	Art. no.
1.	Colour developer CD 2	1.0 pet	D011
2.	Colour developer CD 3	1.0 pet	E013
3.	Colour developer CD 4	1.0 pet	E011
4.	4-Methylaminophenol sulphate (Metol)	1.0 pet	M009
5.	Hydroquinone	1.0 pet	H007
6.	Phenidone	1.0 pet	P004
7.	Hydroxylammonium chloride	0.1 aq	H011
8.	Ammoniumpersulphate	2.5 pet	A011
9.	Ethylenediamine dihydrochloride	1.0 pet	E005
10.	1H-Benzotriazol	1.0 pet	B006
11.	Glutaraldehyde[s]	0.2 pet	G003
12.	Benzylalcohol	1.0 pet	B008

Serial no.	Substance	Concentration (%)	Art. no.
13.	Hydroxylammonium sulphate[t]	0.1 aq	H012
14.	Potassium dichromate[t]	0.5 pet	P014
15.	4-Amino-*N,N*-diethylaniline sulphate (TSS)	1.0 pet	A007
16.	Tricresyl phosphate	5.0 pet	T015

[r]Revised May 1993.

[s]Also present in standard series.

[t]Emulsified with sorbitan sesquioleate 5%.

Plant series[u]

Serial no.	Substance	Concentration (%)	Art. no.
1.	*Chamomilla romana* e) (Anthemis nobilis)	1.0 pet	C029
2.	Diallyldisulphide	1.0 pet	D048
3.	*Arnica montana* e) (Mountain tobacco)	0.5 pet	A024
4.	*Taraxacum officinale* e) (Dandelion)	2.5 pet	T032
5.	*Achillea millefolium* e) (Yarrow)	1.0 pet	A025
6.	*Propolis*	10.0 pet	P022
7.	*Chrysanthemum cinerariaefolium* e) (Pyrethrum)	1.0 pet	C031
8.	Sesquiterpene lactone mix[v]	0.1 pet	Mx18
9.	α-Methylene-γ-butyrolactone	0.01 pet	M026
10.	*Tanacetum vulgare* e) (Tansy)	1.0 pet	T033
11.	Alantolactone	0.1 pet	A003
12.	Lichen acid mix:	0.3 pet	Mx15
	Atranorin	0.1 pet	
	Usnic acid	0.1 pet	
	Evernic acid	0.1 pet	
13.	Parthenolide	0.1 pet	P-029
	e) Plant extract		

[u]Revised May 1997.

[v]Also present in standard series.

Plastics and glues series[w]

Serial no.	Substance	Concentration (%)	Art. no.
1.	Hydroquinone	1.0 pet	H007
2.	Dibutyl phthalate	5.0 pet	D007
3.	Phenyl salicylate	1.0 pet	P011
4.	Diethylhexylphthalate (Dioctylphthalate)	2.0 pet	D018
5.	2,6-ditert-Butyl-4-cresol (BHT)	2.0 pet	D006
6.	2(2-Hydroxy-5-methylphenyl)benzotriazol	1.0 pet	H016
7.	Benzoylperoxide	1.0 pet	B007
8.	4-tert-Butylcatechol (PTBC)	0.5 pet	B030
9.	Azodiisobutyrodinitrile	1.0 pet	A018
10.	Bisphenol A	1.0 pet	B013
11.	Tricresyl phosphate	5.0 pet	T015
12.	Phenol formaldehyde resin (P-F-R-2)	1.0 pet	P005
13.	*p*-tert-Butylphenol formaldehyde resin[x]	1.0 pet	B024
14.	Triphenyl phosphate	5.0 pet	T022
15.	Toluenesulphonamide formaldehyde resin	10.0 pet	T010
16.	Resorcinol monobenzoate	1.0 pet	R002
17.	2-Phenylindole	2.0 pet	P007
18.	2-tert-Butyl-4-methoxyphenol (BHA)	2.0 pet	B022

Serial no.	Substance	Concentration (%)	Art. no.
19.	Abitol	10.0 pet	A002
20.	4-tert-Butylphenol	1.0 pet	B023
21.	2-Monomethylol phenol	1.0 pet	M015
22.	Diphenyl thiourea	1.0 pet	D025
23.	2-n-Octyl-4-isothiazolin-3-one	0.1 pet	O004
24.	Cyclohexanone resin	1.0 pet	C027
25.	Triglycidyl isocyanurate	0.5 pet	T028

[w]Revised May 1990.

[x]Also present in standard series.

Rubber additives series

Serial no.	Substance	Concentration (%)	Art. no.
1.	Tetramethylthiuram disulphide	1.0 pet	T005
2.	Tetramethylthiuram monosulphide	1.0 pet	T006
3.	Tetraethylthiuram disulphide	1.0 pet	T002
4.	Dipentamethylenethiuram disulphide	1.0 pet	D019
5.	*N*-Cyclohexyl-*N*-phenyl-4-phenylenediamine	1.0 pet	C024
6.	*N,N*-Diphenyl-4-phenylenediamine[y]	1.0 pet	D024
7.	*N*-Isopropyl-*N*-phenyl-4-phenylenediamine[y]	0.1 pet	I004
8.	2-Mercaptobenzothiazole[y]	2.0 pet	M003
9.	*N*-Cyclohexylbenzothiazyl sulphenamide	1.0 pet	C023
10.	Dibenzothiazyl disulphide	1.0 pet	D003
11.	Morpholinylmercapto benzothiazole	1.0 pet	M016
12.	Diphenylguanidine	1.0 pet	D022
13.	Zinc diethyldithiocarbamate	1.0 pet	Z003
14.	Zinc dibutyldithiocarbamate	1.0 pet	Z002
15.	*N,N*-Di-beta-naphtyl-4-phenylenediamine	1.0 pet	D017
16.	*N*-Phenyl-2-naphtylamine	1.0 pet	P009
17.	Hexamethylenetetramine	2.0 pet	H003
18.	Diaminodiphenylmethane	0.5 pet	D001
19.	Diphenylthiourea	1.0 pet	D025
20.	Zinc dimethyldithiocarbamate	1.0 pet	Z004
21.	2,2,4-Trimethyl-1,2-dihydroquinoline	1.0 pet	T020
22.	Diethylthiourea	1.0 pet	D039
23.	Dibutylthiourea	1.0 pet	D038
24.	Dodecylmercaptan	0.1 pet	D043

[y]Also present in standard series.

Photopatch[z]

Serial no.	Substance	Concentration (%)	Art. no.
1.	Trichlorocarbanilide (TCC)	1.0 pet	T013
2.	Promethazine hydrochloride	1.0 pet	P017
3.	4-Aminobenzoic acid (PABA)	5.0 pet	A006
4.	Tribromsalicylanilide (TBS)	1.0 pet	T012
5.	Chlorpromazine hydrochloride	0.1 pet	C011
6.	2-Hydroxy-4-methoxybenzophenone (Eusolex 4360, Escalol 567, Oxybenzone)	2.0 pet	H014
7.	6-Methylcoumarine (6-MC)	1.0 pet	M010
8.	Bithionol	1.0 pet	B014

Serial no.	*Substance*	*Concentration (%)*	*Art. no.*
9.	Fentichlor	1.0 pet	F001
10.	(+)-Usnic acid	0.1 pet	U005
11.	Atranorin	0.1 pet	A016
12.	Wood mix (pine, spruce, birch, teak)	20.0 pet	Mx09
13.	Evernic acid	0.1 pet	E017
14.	Balsam of Peru[aa]	25.0 pet	B001
15.	Tetrachlorsalicylanilide (TCS)	0.1 pet	T001
16.	Hexachlorophene	1.0 pet	H001
17.	Chlorhexidine digluconate	0.5 aq	C005
18.	Triclosan (Irgasan DP 300)	2.0 pet	T014
19.	Diphenhydramine hydrochloride	1.0 pet	D021
20.	Perfume mix:	6.0 pet	Mx08
	Cinnamic alcohol	1.0	C013
	Cinnamic aldehyde	1.0	C014
	Hydroxycitronellal	1.0	H008
	Eugenol	1.0	E016
	Isoeugenol	1.0	I002
	Geraniol	1.0	G001

[z]Revised October 1997.

[aa]Also present in standard series.

Shoe series[bb]

1.	*N*-Isopropyl-*N*-phenyl-4-phenylenediamine[cc]	0.1 pet	I004
2.	Glutaraldehyde[dd]	0.2 pet	G003
3.	Disperse Orange 3	1.0 pet	D032
4.	acid yellow 36	1.0 pet	A019
5.	Hydroquinone monobenzylether	1.0 pet	H019
6.	Thiuram mix[cc]	1.0 pet	Mx01
7.	Potassium dichromate[cc]	0.5 pet	P014
8.	4-tert-Butylphenol formaldehyde resin[cc]	1.0 pet	B024
9.	4-Phenylenediamine base[cc]	1.0 pet	P006
10.	Nickel sulphate[cc]	5.0 pet	N002
11.	Colophony[cc]	20.0 pet	C020
12.	Formaldehyde[cc]	1.0 aq	F002
13.	Diphenyl thiourea	1.0 pet	D025
14.	2-Mercaptobenzothiazole	2.0 pet	M003
15.	Diethylthiourea	1.0 pet	D039
16.	Diphenylguanidine	1.0 pet	D022
17.	Dibutylthiourea	1.0 pet	D038
18.	Epoxy resin[cc]	1.0 pet	E002
19.	Dodecylmercaptan	0.1 pet	D043
20.	Cl+Me-isothiazolinone[cc] (Kathon CG,200 ppm)	0.02 aq	C009B
21.	4-Aminoazobenzene	0.25 pet	A005
22.	2-n-Octyl-4-isothiazolin-3-one	0.1 pet	O004

[bb]Revised May 1993.

[cc]Also present in standard series.

[dd]Emulsified with sorbitan sesquioleate 5%.

Serial no.	Substance	Concentration (%)	Art. no.
Sunscreen series[ee]			
1.	4-tert-Butyl-4'-methoxy-dibenzoylmethane (Parsol 1789)	2.0 pet	B029
2.	4-Aminobenzoic acid (PABA)	5.0 pet	A006
3.	4-Isopropyl-dibenzoylmethane (Eusolex 8020)	2.0 pet	I005
4.	3-(4-Methylbenzyliden)camphor (Eusolex 6300)	2.0 pet	M024
5.	2-Ethylhexyl-4-dimethylaminobenzoate (Eusolex 6007, Escalol 507, Octyl Dimethyl-PABA)	2.0 pet	E018
6.	2-Hydroxy-4-methoxybenzophenone (Eusolex 4360, Escalol 567, Oxybenzone)	2.0 pet	H014
7.	2-Ethylhexyl-4-methoxycinnamate (Parsol MCX, Escalol 557)	2.0 pet	E019
8.	2-Hydroxy-methoxymethylbenzophenone (Mexenone)	2.0 pet	H020
9.	2-Phenylbenzimidazol-5-sulphonic acid (Eusolex 232, Novantisol)	2.0 pet	P024
10.	2-Hydroxy-4-methoxybenzophenon-5-sulphonic acid (Sulisobenzone, Uvinyl MS-40, Benzophenone 4)	5.0 pet	H023

[ee]Revised August 1992.

[ff]Important series to be used in photopatch testing.

Serial no.	Substance	Concentration (%)	Art. no.
Textile colours and finish[gg]			
1.	Disperse yellow 3	1.0 pet	D036
2.	Disperse orange 3	1.0 pet	D032
3.	Disperse red 1	1.0 pet	D034
4.	Disperse red 17	1.0 pet	D035
5.	Disperse blue 153	1.0 pet	D029
6.	Disperse blue 3	1.0 pet	D026
7.	Disperse blue 35	1.0 pet	D027
8.	Dimethylol dihydroxyethyleneurea (Fix.CPN)	4.5 aq	D012
9.	Dimethylol propylene urea (Fix.PH)	5.0 aq	D014
10.	Tetramethylol acetylenediurea (Fix.140)	5.0 aq	T003
11.	Disperse blue 106	1.0 pet	D040
12.	Ethyleneurea, melamineformaldehyde (Fix.Ac)[hh]	5.0 pet	Mx16
13.	Urea formaldehyde (Kaurit S)	10.0 pet	U001
14.	Melamine formaldehyde (Kaurit M70)	7.0 pet	M001
15.	Disperse blue 85	1.0 pet	D028
16.	Disperse orange 1	1.0 pet	D031
17.	Disperse orange 13	1.0 pet	D033
18.	Disperse brown 1	1.0 pet	D030
19.	Disperse yellow 9	1.0 pet	D037

Serial no.	*Substance*	*Concentration (%)*	*Art. no.*
20.	Disperse blue 124	1.0 pet	D041
21.	Basic red 46	1.0 pet	B026

[gg]Revised May 1997.

[hh]Emulsified with sorbitan sesquioleate 5%.

Various allergens[ii]

1.	Prilocaine hydrochloride	5.0 pet	P027
2.	Ammonium tetrachloroplatinate	0.25 aq	A013
3.	Ammonium hexachloroplatinate	0.1 aq	A010
4.	Olive oil	100	O006
5.	Tetramethylbenzidine	0.1 pet	T004
6.	EDTA	1.0 pet	E006
7.	Nigrosin	1.0 pet	N003
8.	Musk mix (xylene, tibetine, moskene, ketone)	4.0 pet	Mx10
9.	Cadmium chloride	1.0 aq	C001
10.	Ethoxyquin	0.5 pet	E003
11.	Chlorhexidine diacetate	0.5 aq	C004
12.	Oleamidopropyl dimethylamine	0.1 aq	O005
13.	Zinc	2.5 pet	Z001
14.	Copper oxide	5.0 pet	C021
15.	Mercuric chloride	0.1 pet	M004
16.	Coal tar	5.0 pet	C016
17.	White petrolatum (Penreco Snow White)	100	P003
18.	Clioquinol (Chinoform, Vioform)	5.0 pet	C015
19.	Chlorquinaldol (Sterosan)	5.0 pet	C012
20.	Methyl-4-hydroxybenzoate	3.0 pet	M012
21.	Ethyl-4-hydroxybenzoate	3.0 pet	E010
22.	Propyl-4-hydroxybenzoate	3.0 pet	P020
23.	Butyl-4-hydroxybenzoate	3.0 pet	B020
24.	Benzyl-4-hydroxybenzoate	3.0 pet	B009
25.	Pine tar	3.0 pet	P012
26.	Beech tar	3.0 pet	B002
27.	Juniper tar	3.0 pet	J003
28.	Birch tar	3.0 pet	B011
29.	Procaine hydrochloride	1.0 pet	P016
30.	Dibucaine hydrochloride	5.0 pet	D005
31.	Naphtyl mix (DBNPD 0.5%, PBN 0.5%)	1.0 pet	Mx11
32.	4-Aminoazobenzene	0.25 pet	A005
33.	Turpentine peroxides	0.3 o.o.	T024
34.	Caine mix I:	3.5 pet	
	Procaine-HC	1.0 pet	
	Dibucaine-HCl	2.5 pet	Mx12
35.	Wood tar mix (pine, beech, juniper, birch)	12.0 pet	Mx14
36.	Caine mix II:	10.0 pet	Mx13
	Dibucaine–HCl	2.5 pet	
	Lidocaine	5.0 pet	
	Tetracaine–HCl	2.5 pet	

Serial no.	Substance	Concentration (%)	Art. no.
37.	Cobalt chloride	0.5 pet	C017B
38.	Deleted		
39.	4-Phenylenediamine dihydrochloride	0.5 pet	P028
40.	Ethyleneurea	1.0 pet	E008
41.	Silver nitrate	1.0 aq	S007
42.	Tetracaine hydrochloride	5.0 pet	T025
43.	Balsam of Tolu	10.0 alc	B025
44.	Styrax	2.0 pet	S008
45.	Amylocaine hydrochloride	5.0 pet	A020
46.	Benzalkonium chloride	0.1 aq	B027
47.	Mercury ammonium chloride	1.0 pet	M022
48.	Thiourea	0.1 pet	T026
49.	Potassium dicyanoaurate	0.1 aq	P015
50.	Aluminum	100	A021
51.	Lidocaine	5.0 pet	L002
52.	Carba mix(DPG+ZBC+ZDC)	3.0 pet	Mx06
53.	Black rubber mix:	0.6 pet	Mx04
	N-Isopropyl-*N*-phenyl-4-phenylenediamine	0.1	I004
	N-Cyclohexyl-*N*-phenyl-4-phenylene-diamine	0.25	C024
	N,N-Diphenyl-4-phenylenediamine	0.25	D024

[ii]Revised October 1997.

Aeroallergen patch tests[jj]

1.	Dermatophagoides mix (vol = 2.5ml) (Pteronyssinus/Pharinae)[kk]	40 pet	Mx21
2.	Dermatophagoides mix (vol = 2.5ml) (Pteronyssinus/Pharinae)[kk]	20 pet	Mx21B

[jj]Revised October 1997.

[kk]Divergent price, ask for quotation.

Thiuram mix	1.0 pet	Mx-01 S,SH
Tetramethylthiuram monosulphide		
Tetramethylthiuram disulphide		
Tetraethylthiuram disulphide		
Dipentamethylenethiuram disulphide		
Quinoline mix	6.0% pet	Mx-02 S
Clioquinol		
Chlorquinaldol		
Parabens	12.0 pet	Mx-03 C,S
Methyl-4-hydroxybenzoate		
Ethyl-4-hydroxybenzoate		
Propyl-4-hydroxybenzoate		
Butyl-4-hydroxybenzoate		

Serial no.	*Substance*	*Concentration (%)*	*Art. no.*
	Black rubber mix	0.6 pet	Mx-04 V
	N-Isopropyl-*N*-phenyl-4-phenylenediamine		
	N-Cyclohexyl-*N*-phenyl-4-phenylenediamine		
	N,N-Diphenyl-4-phenylenediamine		
	Mercapto mix	2.0 pet	Mx-05 S
	N-cyclohexylbenzothiazyl sulphenamide		
	Mercaptobenzothiazole		
	Dibenzothiazyl disulphide		
	Morpholinylmercaptobenzothiazole		
	Carba mix	3.0% pet	Mx-06 V
	1,3-Diphenylguanidine		
	Zinc diethyldithiocarbamate		
	Zinc dibutyldithiocarbamate		
	Fragrance mix[ll]	8.0 pet	Mx-07 S
	Cinnamic alcohol		
	Cinnamic aldehyde		
	Hydroxycitronellal		
	Amylcinnamaldehyde		
	Geraniol		
	Eugenol		
	Isoeugenol		
	Oakmoss absolute		

[ll]Emulsifier: sorbitan sesquioleate 5%.

Serial no.	*Substance*	*Concentration (%)*	*Art. no.*
	Perfume mix	6.0 pet	Mx-08 SP
	Cinnamic alcohol		
	Cinnamic aldehyde		
	Hydroxycitronellal		
	Eugenol		
	Isoeugenol		
	Geraniol		
	Wood mix	20.0 pet	Mx-09 SP
	Pine		
	Spruce		
	Birch		
	Teak		
	Musk mix	4.0 pet	Mx-10 V
	Musk xylene		
	Musk tibetine		
	Musk ketone		
	Musk moskene		
	Naphtyl mix	1.0 pet	Mx-11 V
	N,N-Di-beta-naphtyl-4-phenylenediamine		
	N-Phenyl-2-naphtylamine		

Serial no.	Substance	Concentration (%)	Art. no.
	Caine mix I	3.5 pet	Mx-12 V
	Procaine hydrochloride		
	Dibucaine hydrochloride		
	Caine mix II	10.0 pet	Mx-13 V
	Dibucaine hydrochloride		
	Lidocaine		
	Tetracaine hydrochloride		
	Wood tar mix	12.0 pet	Mx-14 V
	Pine		
	Beech		
	Juniper		
	Birch		
	Lichen acid mix	0.3 pet	Mx-15 PL
	Atranorin		
	Evernic acid		
	D-Usnic acid		
	Ethyleneurea, melamine-formaldehyde mix	5.0 pet	Mx-16 TF
	Ethyleneurea		
	Melamineformaldehyde		
	Euxyl K 400	0.5 pet	Mx-17 C,O
	1,2-Dibromo-2,4-dicyanobutane		
	2-Phenoxyethanol		
	Sesquiterpene lactone mix	0.1 pet	Mx-18 S,PL
	Alantolactone		
	Dehydrocostus lactone		
	Costunolide		
	Caine mix III	10.0 pet	Mx-19 ME
	Benzocaine		
	Cinchocaine (dibucaine)		
	Tetracaine (amethocaine)		
	Caine mix IV	10.0 pet	Mx-20 ME
	Amylocaine hydrochloride		
	Lignocaine (lidocaine)		
	Prilocaine (propitocaine)		
	Dermatophagoides mix[mm]		Mx-21 SA
		(40 & 20)	Mx-21B SA
	Pteronyssinus		
	Pharinae		

[mm]Volume = 2.5 ml.

Brial Allergens

Substance	Concentration (%)	Art. no.
European standard		
Potassium dichromate	0.5 pet	0001
p-Phenylenediamine free base	1 pet	0305
Thiuram mix	1 pet	0003
Neomycin sulphate	20 pet	0004
Cobalt chloride	1 pet	0005
Benzocaine	5 pet	0006
Nickel sulphate	5 pet	0007/1
Colophony	20 pet	0308
Paraben-mix	16 pet	0010/1
IPPD	0.1 pet	0915
Wool alcohols	30 pet	0012
Mercapto mix	1 pet	0013/1
Epoxy resin	1 pet	0014/1
Balsam of Peru	25 pet	0015
p-tert-Butylphenol-formaldehyde resin	1 pet	0016
Formaldehyde	1 aq	0018
Fragrance mix	8 pet	0019
2-Mercaptobenzothiazole	2 pet	0022
(Cl)-Methylisothiazolinone	0.01 aq	1013
Petrolatum	100	1600
Ammoniated mercury	1 pet	1301
Cetylstearylalcohol	20 pet	1604
Bis-(diethyldithiocarbamato)-zinc	1 pet	0911
Thimerosal	0.1 pet	1300
Dibromdicyanobutan/phenoxyethanol (1:4)	0.5 pet	1021
Venice turpentine	10 pet	0701
Supplementary recommendation:		
Ethylenediamine–HCl	1 pet	0020/1
Quaternium 15	1 pet	0021
Chlorquinaldol	5 pet	0026
1,3-Diphenylguanidine	1 pet	0905
Topical medicaments		
Chloramphenicol	2 pet	1101
Tetracycline–HCl	2 pet	1102
Kanamycin sulphate	10 pet	1103
Gentamicin sulphate	20 pet	1104
Ampicillin	5 pet	1105
Streptomycin sulphate	5 pet	1107
Bacitracin	20 pet	1111/1
Bufexamac	5 pet	1831
Quinine sulphate	25 pet	2201

Substance	*Concentration (%)*	*Art. no.*
Mafenide	10 pet	1414
Methyl salicylate	2 pet	2008
Sulphur precipitated	10 pet	1805
Salicylic acid	5 pet	1806
Procaine–HCl	2 pet	1200
Lidocaine–HCl	15 pet	1203
Tetracaine–HCl	1 pet	1201
Cinchocain–HCl	5 pet	1204
Mepivacaine	1 pet	1205
Clotrimazole	5 pet	1860
Nystatin	2 pet	1862
Dexpanthenol	5 pet	1861
Fusidic acid	2 pet	1113
Polidocanol	3 pet	1863
Propantheline bromide	5 pet	1865
Chlorotetracycline–HCl	1 pet	1106
Oxytetracycline	0.5 pet	1108
Erythromycin	0.5 pet	1109
Sulphanilamide	5 pet	1815/1
Menthol	1 pet	0728
Silver protein	3 pet	1802
Supplementary recommendation:		
Acetylsalicylic acid	10 pet	2200
Aminoantipyrine	10 pet	2202
Phenacetin	10 pet	2203
Phenylbutazone	10 pet	2204
Paracetamol	10 pet	2205
Indomethacin	1 pet	2206
Propyphenazone	1 pet	2207
Metamizol	1 pet	2208
Diclofenac sodium	5 pet	2209
Oxyphenbutazone	10 pet	2210
Atropine sulphate	1 pet	1811
Nitrofurazone	1 pet	1813
Sulphisomidine	10 pet	1814
Adrenaline	1 pet	1818
Sulphathiazole	1 pet	1820
Adiphenine	1 pet	1823
Bibrocathol	2 pet	1824
Naphazoline–HCl	1 pet	1825
Sodium dibunate	1 pet	1826
Salicylamide	2 pet	1827
Citric acid	1 pet	1834
Thiamine nitrate	10 pet	1844
Thiamine–HCl	10 pet	1845
Pyridoxine–HCl	10 pet	1846
Sulphadiazine	2 pet	1852

Substance	Concentration (%)	Art. no.
Metronidazole	1 pet	1854
Penicillamine	1 pet	1855
Caffeine	0.5 pet	1859
Phenyl salicylate	1 pet	1840
Camphor	1 pet	0729
Topical eye medicaments		
Chlorpheniramine maleate	5 pet	0800
Atropine sulphate	1 pet	1811
Iododesoxyuridine	1 pet	5202
Phenylephrine–HCl	10 coca	5203
Cromoglicic disodium salt	2 pet	5205
EDTA–sodium	0.1 pet	5207
Pilocarpine–HCl	1 pet	5210
Papain	1 pet	5216
Cocamidopropylbetain	1 EtOH	0212
Acebutolol–HCl	2 pet	5500
Oxyprenolol–HCl	2 pet	5502
Propanolol–HCl	2 pet	5503
Polymycine-B-sulphate	3 pet	5225
Supplementary recommendation:		
Pindolol	2 pet	5501
Corticosteroids		
Amcinonide	0.1 pet	5600
Budenoside	0.1 pet	5601
Betamethasone-17-valerate	0.12 pet	5602/1
Clobetasol-17-propionate	0.25 pet	5603/1
Dexamethysone	0.5 pet	1819
Hydrocortisone-17-butyrate	0.1 pet	5605/1
Prednisolone	0.5 pet	1821
Hydrocortisone	1 pet	5606
Triamcinolone	0.1 pet	5607
Dental materials		
Triethyleneglycol dimethacrylate	2 pet	2300
Ethyleneglycol dimethacrylate	2 pet	2301
Ammoniumtetrachloroplatinate	0.25 pet	2303
Amalgam metals	20 pet	2350
Amalgam, non gamma 2	5 pet	2351
Copper sulphate	1 aq	2306
Methyl methacrylate	2 pet	2308
Bisphenol A dimethacrylate	2 pet	2309
Bisphenol A	1 pet	0327
Eugenol	1 pet	0401

Substance	*Concentration (%)*	*Art. no.*
2-Hydroxyethyl methacrylate	1 pet	2352
BIS-GMA	2 pet	2353
Urethane dimethacrylate	2 pet	2354
Potassium dicyanoaurate	0.002 pet	2355
Palladium chloride	1 pet	2411
Supplementary recommendation:		
Benzoyl peroxide	1 pet	0101
Tetracaine–HCl	1 pet	1201
Tetrachloroaurate	0.1 pet	2420
Tin-II-chloride	0.5 EtOH	2402
N,N-Dimethyl-*p*-toluidine	2 pet	0326
Preservatives, antimicrobials		
Clioquinol	5 pet	1007
Hexachlorophene	0.5 pet	1002/1
Chlorocresol	1 pet	1004
Benzoic acid	5 pet	1005
Chloroxylenol	1 pet	1006
4-Hexyl-resorcinol	0.25 pet	1008
Chloroacetamide	0.2 pet	1015
Sorbic acid	2 pet	1400
Benzalkonium chloride	0.1 pet	1410
Cetylpyridinium chloride	0.1 pet	1411
Dichlorophene	0.5 pet	1425
Phenoxyethanol	1 pet	1022
tert-Butylhydroquinone	1 pet	1436
Cetalconium chloride	0.1 pet	1437
Chlorhexidine digluconate	0.5 aq	1438
Sodium benzoate	5 pet	1439
2-Hydroxymethyl-2-nitro-1,3-propanediol	1 pet	1442
Zinc pyrithione	0.1 pet	1443
Imidazolidinyl urea	2 pet	1012
Phenylmercuric acetate	0.05 pet	1304
Supplementary recommendation:		
Bronopol	0.5 pet	1014
Methyl-*p*-hydroxybenzoate	3 pet	1401
Propyl-*p*-hydroxybenzoate	3 pet	1402
Butyl-*p*-hydroxybenzoate	3 pet	1403
Ethyl-*p*-hydroxybenzoate	3 pet	1405
Glutaraldehyde	0.3 pet	1409/1
Benzotriazole	1 pet	1416
Triclosan	2 pet	1417
Butylhydroxytoluene	2 pet	1419
Butylhydroxyanisole	2 pet	1420
Dodecyl gallate	0.3 pet	1431

Substance	*Concentration (%)*	*Art. no.*
Octyl gallate	0.3 pet	1432
Propyl gallate	0.5 pet	1433
DMDM Hydantoin	2 pet	1435
Benzisothiazolinone	0.1 pet	1023
Diazolidinyl urea	2 pet	1024
Phenylmercuric nitrate	0.01 pet	1308
Iodine	0.5 pet	1408
Perfumes and flavours		
Turpentine	10 pet	0740
Oil of eucalyptus	2 pet	0407
Oil of cloves	2 pet	0413
Benzyl alcohol	1 pet	0423/1
Vanillin	10 pet	0438
Oil of laurel	2 pet	0439
Oil of peppermint	2 pet	0440
Oil neroli	2 pet	0444
Salicylaldehyde	2 pet	0435
Oil cedar	10 pet	0445
Benzaldehyde	5 pet	0436
Cinnamic acid	5 pet	0446
Benzylsalicylate	1 pet	0447
Eugenol	1 pet	0401
Citronellal	2 pet	0400
Supplementary recommendation:		
Cinnamon oil	0.5 pet	0100
D-Limonene	2 pet	0104/1
Geraniol	1 pet	0403
Cinnamic aldehyde	1 pet	0404/1
Cinnamic alcohol	1 pet	0424
Isoeugenol	1 pet	0427
Oak moss absolute	2 pet	0428
Hypericon oil	0.5 pet	0408
Oil of rose	0.5 pet	0410
Oil of rosemary	0.5 pet	0411
Oil of lemon	0.5 pet	0412
Amyl cinnamic aldhyde	1 pet	0425
Hydroxycitronellal	1 pet	0426
Coumarin	1 pet	0429
Oil of lemon grass	2 pet	0433
Oil of bergamot	2 pet	0441
Orange oil	2 pet	0448
Dyes		
4-Aminoazobenzene	0.25 pet	0600
Disperse yellow 3	1 pet	0603

Substance	Concentration (%)	Art. no.
Disperse orange 3	1 pet	0604
Disperse blue 3	1 pet	0610
4-Aminophenol	1 pet	0612
Disperse red 1	1 pet	0614
Disperse blue 106	1 pet	0620
Disperse red 11	1 pet	0621
Disperse yellow 9	1 pet	0622
Disperse blue 1	1 pet	0624
Disperse red 17	1 pet	0625
Metanil yellow	1 pet	0626
p-Aminodiphenylamine	0.25 pet	0200
Vesuvine brown	0.5 pet	0627
Naphthol-AS	1 pet	0623
Supplementary recommendation:		
Methyl viole	0.5 pet	0607
Erythrosine-B	0.25 pet	0609
Eosine-g	50 pet	0613
Phenolphthalein	0.5 pet	0619
Aniline	1 pet	0601
Photoallergens		
Chlorpromazine–HCl	1 pet	1904
Promethazine–HCl	2 pet	1906
Frusemide	1 pet	1908
Chlorphenoxamine–HCl	1 pet	1911
Sulphanilamide	5 pet	1815/1
Musk ambrette	5 pet	0443
Tribromsalan	1 pet	1920
Chinidinum sulphuricum	1 pet	1864
Phenylbenzimidazolesulphonic acid	10 pet	2014
Thiourea	0.1 pet	0209
Bithionol	1 pet	1001
Hexachlorophene	1 pet	1002
Alimaemazine tartrate	1 pet	0804
3,4,4'-Triclocarban	1 pet	1428
Olaquindox	1 pet	1921
Photographic chemicals		
Methylaminophenolsulphate	1 pet	0501
Hydrazine sulphate	1 pet	0502
Colour developer CD 3	1 pet	0503
Colour developer CD 4	1 pet	0504
1-Phenyl-3-pyrazolidinone	1 pet	0505
Triphenyl phosphate	5 pet	0323
4-Aminophenol	2 pet	0612
Hydroquinone	1 pet	0304

Substance	*Concentration (%)*	*Art. no.*
Pyrogallol	1 pet	0207
Ammonium persulphate	2.5 pet	0102/1
Hairdressing		
o-Nitro-*p*-phenylenediamine	1 pet	0201
Resorcinol	1 pet	0202/1
p-Toluenediamine sulphate	1 pet	0203
Pyrogallol	1 pet	0207
Ammmonium thioglycolate	1 pet	0208/1
Glyceryl monothioglycolate	1 pet	0210
Ammonium persulphate	2.5 pet	0102/1
4-Aminophenol	1 pet	0612
3-Aminophenol	1 pet	0211
Cocamidopropylbetaine	1 aq/EtOH	0212
Rubber chemicals		
Hexamethylenetetramine	1 pet	0909
Bis(dibuthyldithiocarbamato)–zinc	1 pet	0912
N-Phenyl-β-naphthylamine	1 pet	0913
4,4'-Dihydroxybiphenyl	0.1 pet	0925
Diphenyl-*p*-phenylenediamine	0.25 pet	0025
Cyclohexyl thiophthalimid	1 pet	0932
Dibutylthiourea	1 pet	0933
Diphenylthiourea	1 pet	0934
2-Mercaptobenzimidazole	1 pet	0914
Hydroquinone monobenzylether	1 pet	0922
Supplementary recommendation:		
N-Cyclohexyl-2-benzothiazyl sulphenamide	1 pet	0903
1,3-Diphenylguanidine	1 pet	0905
Tetraethylthiuram disulphide	0.25 pet	0908
Dibutylphthalate	5 pet	0916
Thiourea	0.1 pet	0209
Tetramethylthiuram monosulphide	0.25 pet	0901
Tetramethylthiuram disulphide	0.25 pet	0023
Dipentamethylenethiuram tetrasulphide	0.25 pet	0920
Dibenzothiazyl disulphide	1 pet	0918
Morpholinomercaptobenzothiazole	1 pet	0919
Sun protectors		
2-Ethylhexyl-*p*-methoxycinnamate	10 pet	2002
4-tert-Butyl-4'-methoxydibenzoylmethane	10 pet	2003
2-Ethylhexyl-4-dimethylaminobenzoate	10 pet	2004
2-Hydroxy-4-methoxybenzophenone	10 pet	2009
4-Isopropyl-dibenzoylmethane	10 pet	2012
2-(4-Methylbenzylidene) camphor	10 pet	2013

Substance	*Concentration (%)*	*Art. no.*
4-Aminobenzoic acid	5 pet	1913
Phenylbenzimidazole sulphonic acid	10 pet	2014
Benzophenone 4	10 pet	2015
Isoamyl-*p*-methoxycinnamate	10 pet	2016
Metal compounds		
Mercury	0.5 pet	1309
Tin (II) chloride	0.5 EtOH	2402
Chromium (III) sulphate	0.5 pet	1833
Ferrous sulphate	5 pet	2405
Silver colloidal	0.1 pet	2415
Zinc powder	1 pet	2416
Copper sulphate	2 pet	2417
Cadmium sulphate	2 pet	2307
Titanium (IV) oxide	0.1 pet	2419
Indium (III) chloride	1 pet	2403/1
Gallium oxide	1 pet	2413
Ammonium heptamolybdate	1 aq	2401
Tantal	1 pet	2311
Tetrachloroaureate	0.1 pet	2420
Potassiumchromate (III) sulphate	2 pet	2421
Supplementary recommendation:		
Palladium chloride	1 pet	2411
Ruthenium	0.1 pet	2414
Ammoniumtertachloroplatinate	0.25 pet	2303
Cobalt (II) sulphate	2.5 pet	0615
Zirconium (IV) oxide	0.1 pet	1019
Zinc chloride	1 pet	2400
Ferrous chloride	2 EtOH	2406/1
Chromium (III) chloride	1 pet	2412
Potassium dicyanoaurate	0.002 pet	2355
Nature substances/household		
D-Limonene	2 pet	0104/1
Turpentine peroxide	0.3 pet	0024
Coal tar	5 pet	0027
Pine tar	3 pet	0703
Ammoniumbituminosulphonate	10 pet	0727
Primin	0.01 pet	0732
Balsam of Tolu	20 pet	0717
Larch turpentine	20 pet	0737
Alpha pinene	15 pet	0707
Propolis	10 pet	0719

Substance	*Concentration (%)*	*Art. no.*
Supplementary recommendation:		
Benzoe tincture	10 EtOH	0702
Atranorin	0.1 pet	0713
Usnic acid	0.1 pet	0714
Wood tars mix	12 pet	1703
Sesquiterpene lactone mix	0.1 pet	0733
Pesticides		
Captan	0.1 pet	1505
Malathion	0.5 pet	1513
Maneb	1 pet	1516
Zineb	1 pet	1517
Pyrethrum	2 pet	1519
Captafol	0.1 pet	1520
Benomyl	0.1 pet	1521
Folpet	0.1 pet	1522
Lindane	0.5 pet	1504
Plastic and glues		
Benzoyl peroxide	1 pet	0101
Butylacrylate	0.1 pet	0205
2-Ethylhexyl acrylate	0.1 pet	0206
Dimethylphthalate	5 pet	0311
Dibutylphthalate	5 pet	0916
4,4-Diaminodiphenyl methane	0.5 pet	0313
Resorcinol-formaldehyde resin	5 pet	0314
Phenol-formaldehyde resin	5 pet	0315
Triethylenetetramine	0.5 pet	0316
p-tert-Butylphenol	1 pet	0318
Diethylphthalate	5 pet	0320
Phenylisocyanate	0.1 pet	0322
N,N-Dimethyl-*p*-toluidine	2 pet	0326
Abietic acid	5 pet	0328
Tricresyl phosphate	5 pet	0329
4-tert-Butylcatchol	1 pet	0338
Bis-(2-ethylhexyl)phthalate	5 pet	0324
Isophrorone diamine	0.5 pet	0332
o-Cresyl glycidyl ether	0.25 pet	0335
Diphenylmethane-4,4-diisocyanate	0.1 pet	0336
Supplementary recommendation:		
Triethylenediamine	0.5 pet	0301
Diethylenetetramine	0.5 pet	0317
Triphenyl phosphate	5 pet	0323
Toluenesulphonamide formaldehyde resin	10 pet	0331
Epichlorhydrin	0.1 pet	0325

Substance	*Concentration (%)*	*Art. no.*
Vehicles and emulsifiers		
Eucerin, anhydrous	100	1602
Cold cream	100	1607
Wool fat	30 pet	1608
Triethanolamine	2.5 pet	1609
Isopropylmyristate	10 pet	1623/1
Propylene glycol	5 pet	1624
Polyethylene glycol-400	100	1625
Diachylon	100	1626
Polyethyleneglycol ointment	100	1629
Coconut diethanolamide	0.5 pet	1630
Supplementary recommendation:		
Sorbitan sesquioleate	20 pet	1610
Tween 40	10 pet	1611
Tween 80	10 pet	1612
Amerchol L101	50 pet	1628
Food – additives		
Tatrazine	1 coca	2500
Quinoline yellow	0.1 aq	2501
Carmine	0.5 coca	2503
Azorubine	0.1 aq	2504
Amaranth	0.1 aq	2505
Cochineal red	1 coca	2506
Erythrosin-B	0.25 EtOH	2507
Patent blue VF	0.25 coca	2508
Brilliant black	0.1 aq	2509
Sodium glutamate	1 coca	2511
Saccharine	0.1 coca	2520
Aspartame	0.1 coca	2521
Sodium alginate	1 coca	2530
Pectin-C	1 coca	2531
Sorbic acid	2 EtOH	2540
Benzoic acid	1 EtOH	2541
Sulphur dioxide	2 aq	2545
Sodium sulphite	1 coca	2546
Formic acid	1 aq	2547
Sodium formiate	2 coca	2548
Sodium nitrite	2 aq	2549
Sodium disulphite	1 coca	2550
Sodium diphosphate	1 coca	2560
Butylhydroxyanisole	2 EtOH	2591
Butylhydroxytoluene	1 EtOH	2590

Substance	*Concentration (%)*	*Art. no.*
Composition of the mixes		
Fragrance mix:	8	0019
Eugenol	1 %	0401
Cinnemaic aldehyde	1	0404/1
Cinnemaic alcohol	1	0424
Amylcinnemaic aldehyde	1	0425
Hydroxycitronellal	1	0426
Isoeugenol	1	0427
Oak moss absolute	1	0428
Wood tars mix:	12	1703
Birch tar	3	
Juniper tar	3	
Beech tar	3	
Canadian balsam	3	
Parabens mix:	16	0010/1
Methyl-*p*-hydroxybenzoate	4	1401
Propyl-*p*-hydroxybenzoate	4	1402
Butyl-*p*-hydroxybenzoate	4	1403
Ethyl-*p*-hydroxybenzoate	4	1405
Mercapto mix:	1	0013/1
N-Cyclohexyl-2-benzothiazylsulphenamide	0.333	0903
Dibenzothiazyldisulphide (DBTS)	0.333	0918
Morpholinomercapobenzothiazole (MMBT)	0.333	0919
Thiuram mix:	1	0003
Tetramethylthiurammonosulphide (TMTM)	0.25	0901
Tetramethyldisulphide (TMTD	0.25	0023
Tetraethylthiuramdisulphide (TETD)	0.25	0908
Dipentamethylenthiuramdisulphide (DPTD)	0.25	

22. Sources of Further Information

Matthias Gebhardt

This book is unable to answer all questions in contact dermatitis. Further reading of review articles, electronic sources of information, books, journals, etc., is highly recommended. Suggested reading includes the following standard books from every dermatology department's library.

1. Rietschel RL, Fowler JFF, eds, *Fisher's contact dermatitis*, 4th edn. Baltimore: Williams & Wilkins; 1995.
2. Cronin E, *Contact dermatitis*. Edinburgh: Churchill Livingstone; 1980.
3. Rycroft RJG, Menne T, Frosch PJ, eds, *Textbook of contact dermatitis*, 2nd edn. Berlin: Springer; 1995.
4. Marks JG Jr, DeLeo VA, *Contact and occupational dermatology*, 2nd edn. St Louis: Mosby; 1997.
5. Guin JD, *Practical contact dermatitis*. McGraw-Hill, 1995.
6. Mitchell J, Rook A, *Botanical dermatology*. Vancouver: Greengrass; 1979. This comprehensive coverage of botanical dermatology has been reorganized by Dr R Schmidt of the University of Cardiff, Wales, and is currently available on the net on <http://bodd.cf.ac.uk>
7. Frosch PJ, Dooms-Goossens A, Lachapelle J-M et al., *Current topics in contact dermatitis*. Heidelberg: Springer; 1989.
8. Hausen BM, Brinkmann J, Dohn W, *Lexikon der Kontaktallergene*. Landsberg/Lech: ecomed Verlagsgesellschaft AG & Co. KG; 1996. An extensive review about several contact allergens for German-speaking readers.
9. De Groot AC, *Patch testing*, 2nd edn. Amsterdam: Elsevier; 1994. The "classic" for patch test concentrations.

Both the journals *Contact Dermatitis* (published by Munksgaard, Copenhagen, Denmark) and *American Journal of Contact Dermatitis* (WB Saunders, Philadelphia) provide continuing information on contact allergy, patch testing, patch test case reports and allergen analysis.

The contact dermatitis homepage offers a great deal of information about contact allergens, allergen providers and references:

<http://www.mc.Vanderbilt.Edu/vumcdept/derm/contact/index.html>

The Botanical Dermatology Database, provided by Richard J Schmidt is available on:

www.uwcm.ac.uk/uwcm/dm/BODD/index-html

INDEX